State-Of-The-Art
Orthodontics

Commissioning Editor: *Alison Taylor*

Development Editor: *Barbara Simmons*

Project Manager: *Nancy Arnott*

Designer: *Stewart Larking*

Illustration Manager: *Gillian Richards*

STATE-OF-THE-ART
ORTHODONTICS

SELF-LIGATING APPLIANCES, MINISCREWS
AND **SECOND MOLAR EXTRACTIONS**

HUGO TREVISI

Orthodontist, Presidente Prudente, Brazil

REGINALDO TREVISI ZANELATO

Orthodontist, Presidente Prudente, Brazil

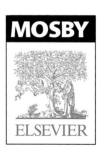

EDINBURGH LONDON NEW YORK OXFORD PHILADELPHIA ST LOUIS SYDNEY TORONTO 2011

MOSBY
ELSEVIER

An imprint of Elsevier Limited

ISBN 9780723436539

British Library Cataloguing in Publication Data
A catalogue record for this book is available from the British Library

Library of Congress Cataloging in Publication Data
A catalog record for this book is available from the Library of Congress

Notices

Knowledge and best practice in this field are constantly changing. As new research and experience broaden our understanding, changes in research methods, professional practices, or medical treatment may become necessary.

Practitioners and researchers must always rely on their own experience and knowledge in evaluating and using any information, methods, compounds, or experiments described herein. In using such information or methods they should be mindful of their own safety and the safety of others, including parties for whom they have a professional responsibility.

With respect to any drug or pharmaceutical products identified, readers are advised to check the most current information provided (i) on procedures featured or (ii) by the manufacturer of each product to be administered, to verify the recommended dose or formula, the method and duration of administration, and contraindications. It is the responsibility of practitioners, relying on their own experience and knowledge of their patients, to make diagnoses, to determine dosages and the best treatment for each individual patient, and to take all appropriate safety precautions.

To the fullest extent of the law, neither the Publisher nor the authors, contributors, or editors, assume any liability for any injury and/or damage to persons or property as a matter of products liability, negligence or otherwise, or from any use or operation of any methods, products, instructions, or ideas contained in the material herein.

 ELSEVIER your source for books, journals and multimedia in the health sciences

www.elsevierhealth.com

Working together to grow
libraries in developing countries

www.elsevier.com | www.bookaid.org | www.sabre.org

ELSEVIER   BOOK AID International   Sabre Foundation

The publisher's policy is to use **paper manufactured from sustainable forests**

Printed in China

Preface

Current technological advances have had a major impact on contemporary orthodontics, allowing the clinician to provide quality treatment with favorable esthetic results in a shorter time period. Indeed, patients are increasingly seeking orthodontic treatment that does not negatively affect the facial esthetics. Thus, clinicians need to have sound scientific knowledge and appropriate technology at hand to be able to offer optimal treatment to each patient.

The use of esthetic, low-friction orthodontic appliances and orthodontic miniscrews allows faster and more efficient treatment with a reduced risk of the side effects of conventional orthodontic mechanics and tissue damage caused by the orthodontic tooth movement. These appliances also address the issue of lack of cooperation on the part of patients with regard to use of headgear and other traditional intraoral anchorage devices, when treating Class II and Class III malocclusions or severe crowding. Both adolescent and adult patients often refuse to wear these appliances as they are not considered esthetic. This book emphasizes the importance of facial esthetics during orthodontic treatment by describing intraoral anchorage systems that help eliminate the requirement for headgear and also diagnosis, treatment planning and orthodontic biomechanics with second molar extractions. All these are key issues that patients take into consideration when deciding whether or not to undergo orthodontic treatment.

The development of the metal SmartClip™ self-ligating appliance led to the possibility of developing the Clarity™ SL Self-Ligating Appliance. This appliance features the same characteristics as the SmartClip™ self-ligating metal appliance, however, it also fulfills the esthetical needs of patients.

Finally, the book also discusses the concept of second molar extractions in orthodontic treatment. This is a useful option in carefully selected patients in whom the erupting third molars would eventually be a good substitute for the second molars extracted for orthodontic purposes.

Thus this book presents a treatment philosophy based on use of esthetic self-ligating appliances and orthodontic miniscrews for anchorage, and treatment with second molar extraction. All these factors allow the clinician to provide orthodontic treatment with more predictable results and efficient sliding biomechanics with the application of low force levels and more favorable biological responses.

Hugo Trevisi
Reginaldo Trevisi Zanelato

Acknowledgments

Firstly, we wish to thank our wives and our children for their care, understanding and support while we were writing this book. To them, we reattribute with love all these years of being together.

We also want to thank Dr Adriano T. Zanelato, Dr André T. Zanelato, Dr Renata Trevisi, Dr Edson Alves, Dr Cristina Ferro and Dr Fernando Bonini from Brazil, as thanks to their support in daily practice, we were able to collect the scientific material required to write this book.

We acknowledge and very much appreciate the translation work of Michelle Trevisi de Araujo.

Our sincere thanks to our friend Dr Lars Christensen, from England, for his support in revising this book. Lars's work made this book didactic and easy to comprehend.

We also would like to acknowledge our friend David Solid, from Monrovia, USA, for his final revision of the book. Our sincere thanks to Barbara Simmons, Alison Taylor and Nancy Arnott from Elsevier, and Lotika Singha. Thank you for your trust.

Contents

Low-friction esthetic brackets: the Clarity™ SL Self-Ligating Appliance System

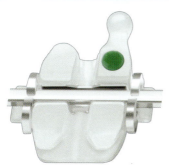

Introduction

A desire for orthodontic treatment that does not adversely affect facial esthetics, both during and after treatment, is increasingly seen in the orthodontic practice. The first esthetic appliances date back to the 1970s and were manufactured in plastic.[1-3]

The Clarity™ appliance, which was released in 1996, had distinctly different characteristics from the other appliances available at that time. The polycrystalline ceramic Clarity™ brackets featured a metal slot, and this bracket design provided excellent facial esthetics with very good sliding biomechanics and precise tridimensional control of teeth during orthodontic treatment. These benefits aimed to fulfill the requirements of an esthetic appliance as could be approved by the orthodontist: that is, it has to allow good torque, tip and rotational control, and be comfortable for the patient. It also has to be easy to place and to remove, exhibit reliable bond strength, and provide a good end result of the orthodontic treatment.

While there are several obvious advantages of esthetic appliances, there are also some disadvantages. One major issue is the change in color of the elastic modules used to hold the archwire in the bracket slot, which is caused by poor oral hygiene or the eating habits of the patient (Figs 1.1, 1.2 & 1.3). The patients

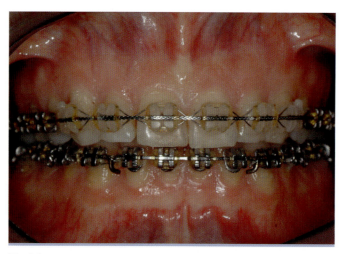

Fig. 1.1

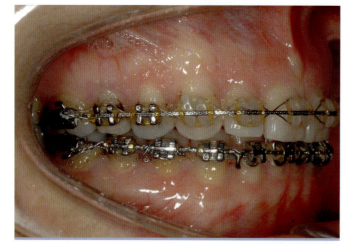

Fig. 1.2

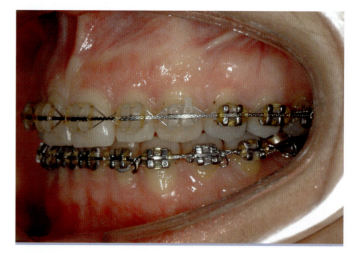

Fig. 1.3

Figs 1.1, 1.2 & 1.3 Change in color of the elastic modules used with conventional appliances, worsening facial esthetics during the course of orthodontic treatment.

who most often experience this problem are those who drink coffee, tea, red wine, etc. on a frequent basis, as well as patients who smoke. These patients have to come back to the office more often simply for new elastic modules in an effort to maintain the esthetics of their appliance.

When the SmartClip™ Self-Ligating Appliance was released in 2004, the possibility of having a Clarity-style appliance featuring the characteristics of a self-ligating appliance became apparent. However, this appliance would not only have to have the same characteristics as the metal[4] self-ligating appliance, but would also have to address the needs of patients who were looking for a more esthetic smile during the treatment. In 2007, new advances in technology made it possible to manufacture the **Clarity™ SL Self-Ligating Appliance**. It featured the same characteristics as the conventional Clarity™ appliance, e.g. a ceramic bracket with a metal slot and a unique debonding mechanism. The Clarity™ SL Self-Ligating Appliance utilizes the same manufacturing technology as the metal self-ligating appliance, with Nitinol clips on the mesial and the distal bracket wings.

Characteristics of the appliance

The Clarity™ SL Self-Ligating Appliance System, which is based on the original concept of the straight-wire appliance, features mid-size, rhomboidal brackets with twin wings. It is a passive bracket system – the archwire is able to slide freely in the bracket slot, with less binding between the wire and the bracket slot when using undersized wires.

The Clarity™ SL Self-Ligating bracket is composed of three parts that are manufactured separately: the ceramic bracket body, the metal slot and the Nitinol clips (Fig. 1.4). The bracket body is manufactured in

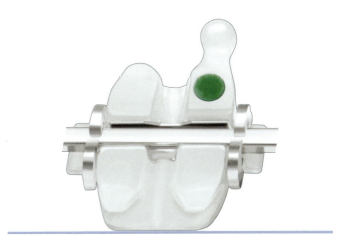

Fig. 1.4 Clarity™ SL Self-Ligating Appliance bracket: note the ceramic bracket body, metal slot and the mesial and distal clips.

ceramics and the bracket slot is produced in metal and inserted in the bracket base. The Nitinol clips are laser cut and pressed onto the mesial and the distal sides of the bracket. The clips are designed to be fatigue resistant while both engaging and removing archwires. As mentioned above, the bracket system offers the same features as the conventional appliance, enabling the use of elastic chains, metal and elastic ligatures and all the other attachments that are usually used with the conventional approach.

The Clarity™ SL Self-Ligating Appliance System prescription

As mentioned above, the Clarity™ SL Self-Ligating Appliance System features a bracket designed for sliding mechanics, that is when using a .019/.025 archwire in the .022/.028 bracket slot. This is usually the last archwire to be used in treatment. The basic orthodontic concepts underlying the use of the Clarity™ SL Self-Ligating Appliance System are the same as those for the SmartClip™ Self-Ligating Appliance System (Figs 1.5, 1.6 & 1.7).

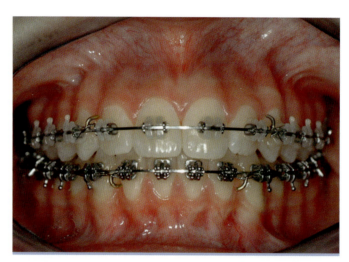

Fig. 1.5

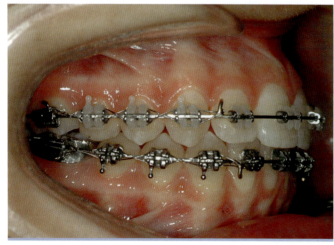

Fig. 1.6

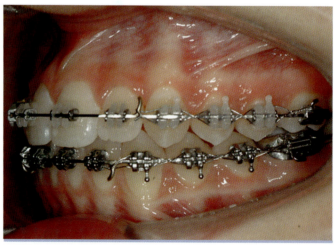

Fig. 1.7

Figs 1.5, 1.6 & 1.7 Clarity™ SL Self-Ligating brackets in the upper arch and the SmartClip™ Self-Ligating Appliance in the lower arch.

Mesiodistal angulation

The basic Clarity™ SL bracket design is the same as the conventional brackets – rhomboidal brackets with built-in angulation. The rhomboidal shape makes bracket positioning easier, along with the use of the individualized bracket positioning system[4–6] (Figs 1.8, 1.9 & 1.10).

The rhomboidal bracket system used with the MBT™ Versatile + Appliance System orthodontic prescription and the individualized bracket positioning system prevents undesirable proclination of the anterior teeth, increased overbite and anchorage loss during the aligning and leveling stages of the orthodontic treatment. The individual bracket positioning system allows positioning of the teeth with due regard to their natural morphology, thus bringing stability to the occlusion that is attained at the end of the treatment.

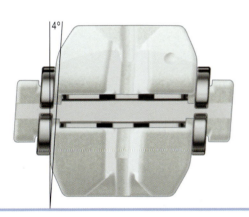

Fig. 1.8 The Clarity™ SL appliance features rhomboidal-shape brackets. This bracket system favors accurate bracket positioning on the facial surface of each tooth.

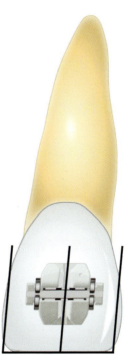

Fig. 1.9 The rhomboidal Clarity™ SL brackets. The bracket is positioned on the facial surface of the clinical crown using the individual bracket positioning line as a reference.

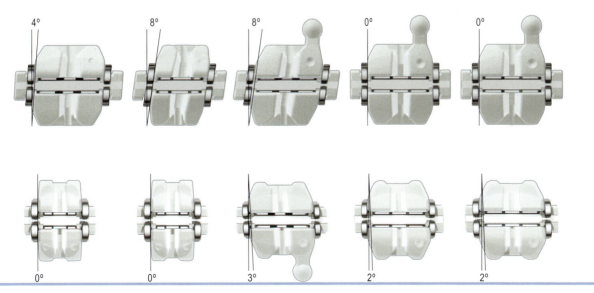

Fig. 1.10 The built-in angulations in the Clarity™ SL Self-Ligating upper and lower brackets.

Inclination (torque)

A highly sophisticated manufacturing process allows the addition of a metal slot into the ceramic bracket body of the Clarity™ SL bracket. The reliability of an orthodontic appliance depends on the degree of expression of the torque that is built into the bracket base and the bracket slot. A metal slot imparts greater strength to the bracket and allows full torque expression. Furthermore, the metal slot facilitates good sliding of the archwire during the orthodontic treatment by reducing friction.[7,8] The Clarity™ SL appliance also features built-in torque in the metal slots (Fig. 1.11).

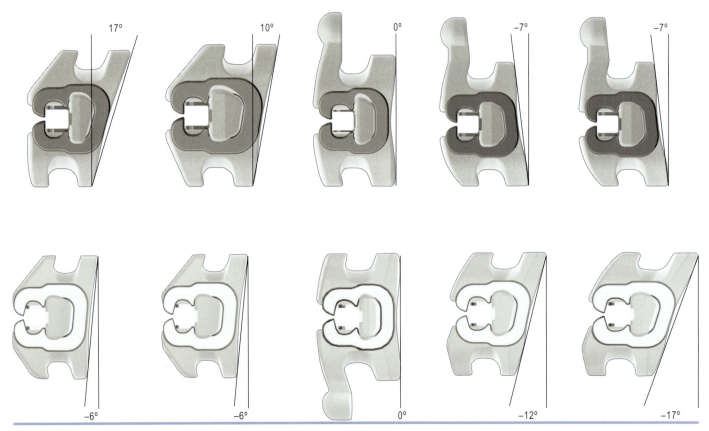

Fig. 1.11 Profile view of the upper and lower Clarity™ SL brackets showing the torque prescriptions.

In-out

From the horizontal aspect, the functional harmony of the orthodontically created occlusion is determined by the in-out built into the appliance, the shapes of the archwires used, and the coordination achieved between the upper and the lower dental arches. The interarch relationships, including the anterior and the canine guidance, and the posterior relationship between the centric cusps and the buccal-occlusal and lingual-occlusal marginal ridges depends on good coordination between the upper and lower arches,[5–8] as well as the in-out prescription of the orthodontic appliance (Figs 1.12 & 1.13). The Clarity™ SL Self-Ligating brackets have been manufactured with this relationship in mind, which allows the simultaneous use of conventional appliances and the SmartClip Self-Ligating appliance in the same patient during orthodontic treatment (see Figs 1.5, 1.6 & 1.7).

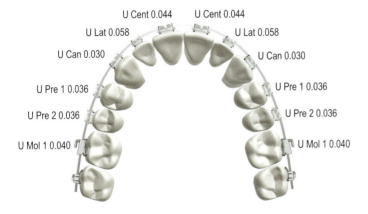

U Cent 0.044   U Cent 0.044
U Lat 0.058   U Lat 0.058
U Can 0.030   U Can 0.030
U Pre 1 0.036 U Pre 1 0.036
U Pre 2 0.036 U Pre 2 0.036
U Mol 1 0.040 U Mol 1 0.040

Fig. 1.12 Occlusal view of the upper arch, showing the in-out prescription of the Clarity™ SL Self-Ligating brackets.

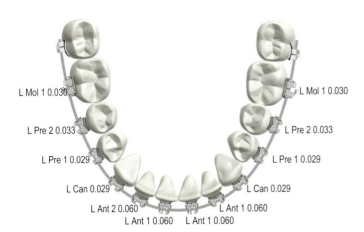

L Mol 1 0.030   L Mol 1 0.030
L Pre 2 0.033   L Pre 2 0.033
L Pre 1 0.029   L Pre 1 0.029
L Can 0.029   L Can 0.029
L Ant 2 0.060   L Ant 1 0.060
L Ant 1 0.060   L Ant 1 0.060

Fig. 1.13 Occlusal view of the lower arch, showing the in-out prescription of the Clarity™ SL Self-Ligating brackets.

Slot depth

As mentioned above, the Clarity™ SL Self-Ligating appliance is a passive appliance, that is, the clip does not exert active pressure on the archwire, unless it is required, e.g. to correct rotations. This allows the use of lower forces during the alignment and the leveling stages of treatment (Figs 1.14, 1.15 & 1.16).[9,10] These stages are completed when the bracket slot is fully filled by the orthodontic archwire in the horizontal plane. The .019/.025 rectangular archwire (Fig. 1.17) or an .016 archwire overlapping the .014 round Nitinol archwire should be engaged on the same visit (see Figs 1.34, 1.35 & 1.36 below).

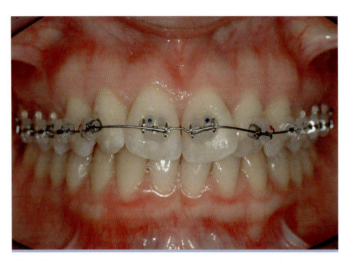

Fig. 1.14

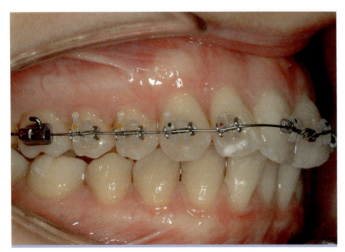

Fig. 1.15

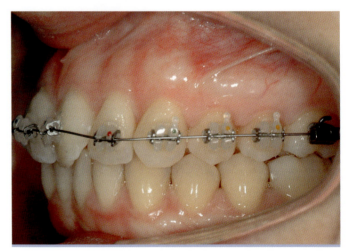

Fig. 1.16

Figs 1.14, 1.15 & 1.16 Initiating the aligning stage with a .014 round Nitinol superelastic wire in the upper arch.

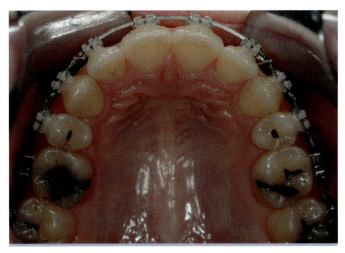

Fig. 1.17 Occlusal view of the upper arch with a .019/.025 rectangular Nitinol archwire in place. Note the good fill of the slot from the horizontal aspect.

The depth of the Clarity™ SL Self-Ligating appliance slot measures .0270 inches between the clip and the bottom of the bracket slot in the lower incisors, and .0275 inches in the remaining teeth. This has been done in order to have improved rotational control at the beginning of treatment (Figs 1.18 & 1.19).

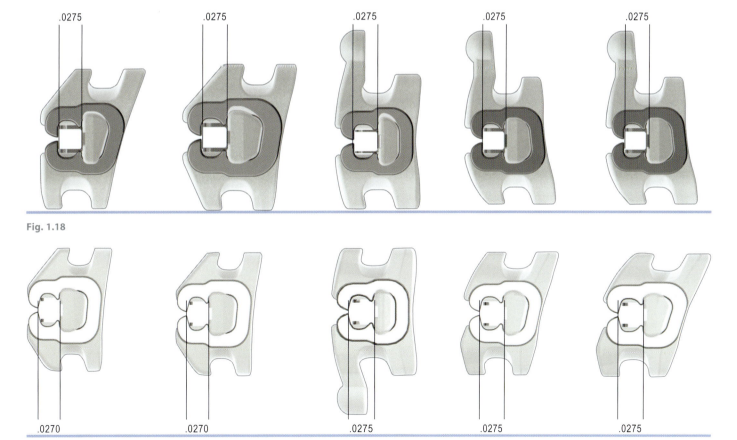

Fig. 1.18

Fig. 1.19

Figs 1.18 & 1.19 Profile views showing the slot-depth between the clip and the bottom of the bracket slot of both upper and lower Clarity™ SL Self-Ligating brackets. Lower incisor brackets have .0270 inch slot depth.

Sliding mechanics with the Clarity™ SL Self-Ligating Appliance

The principle of sliding mechanics[4,5,11,12] can be applied without any need for compromise when using the Clarity™ SL Self-Ligating brackets. The metal slot allows precise accomplishment of aligning, leveling, space closure, and finishing and detailing.

When the orthodontic archwire is allowed to slide freely within the bracket slot in the aligning stages, the masticatory and the muscle forces work in harmony with the applied biomechanics with low force levels, and thus a favorable biological response (Figs 1.20 & 1.21).

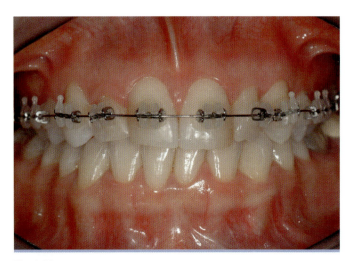

Fig. 1.20

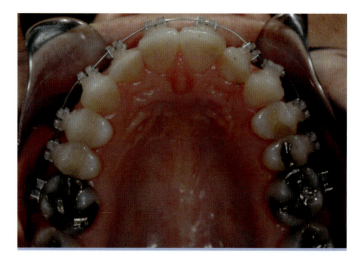

Fig. 1.21

Figs 1.20 & 1.21 Clarity™ SL Self-Ligating Appliance with a .014 round Nitinol superelastic archwire after the initiation of the rotational and the labiolingual corrections.

Aligning

Alignment is the first stage of orthodontic treatment and, depending on the severity of crowding, a .014 round Nitinol or other superelastic archwire can be used regardless of the case being extraction or non-extraction. A .022/.028 bracket provides greater flexibility to .014 archwires, enabling perfect archwire engagement and disengagement using the Nitinol clips (Figs 1.22, 1.23 & 1.24).

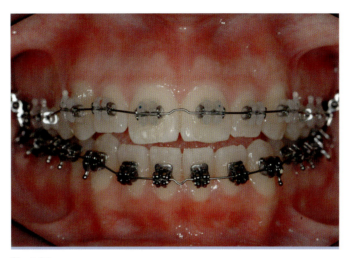

Fig. 1.22

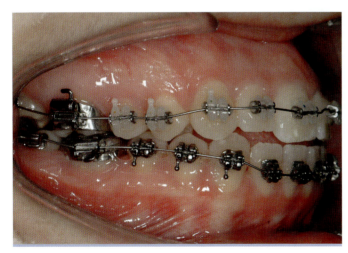

Fig. 1.23

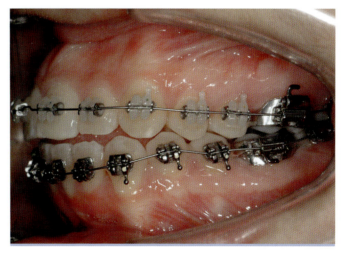

Fig. 1.24

Figs 1.22, 1.23 & 1.24 The .022/.028 Clarity™ SL Self-Ligating Appliance in the upper arch and SmartClip™ Self-Ligating Appliance in the lower arch. An .014 round Nitinol superelastic archwire has been engaged in both the upper and lower dental arches, initiating the alignment stage.

In non-extraction cases, space can be created by proclination or stripping of the incisors, expansion of the intercanine, interpremolar or intermolar width, and distalization or stripping of the posterior teeth. The choice of procedure will depend on the orthodontic treatment plan, incorporating the dental visual treatment objective (dental VTO) analysis.[13]

In premolar extraction cases, the canines should be retracted with lacebacks (which consist of .009 ligature wires), to open up space for the alignment of the incisors (Figs 1.25 & 1.26).

The combination of passive brackets, muscular action and the masticatory function results in biomechanics that favor optimal biological action and tooth movement. In this situation, the initial correction of crowded and malaligned teeth is accomplished faster and with less force application. This stage is frequently finished with a .016 round Nitinol archwire.

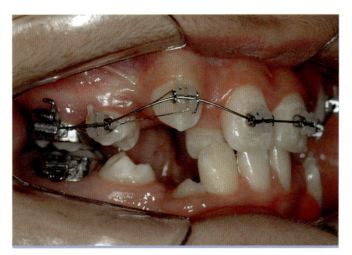

Fig. 1.25

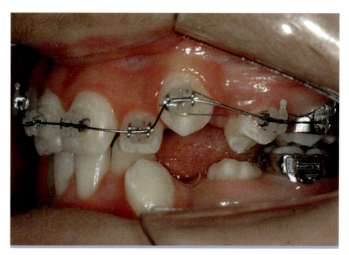

Fig. 1.26

Figs 1.25 & 1.26 Clarity™ SL Self-Ligating appliance in the upper arch, with initiation of canine retraction after premolar extraction.

Leveling

In the leveling stage, the correction of angulations and rotations is completed along with leveling of the bracket slots in the horizontal plane. As mentioned above, space creation in non-extraction cases can be achieved by stripping, proclination of the incisor teeth, distalization of the posterior teeth, and expansion of the intercanine, interpremolar and intermolar widths.

In extraction cases, leveling should be initiated after the retraction of the canines opens up spaces for the alignment of the incisors (Figs 1.27, 1.28, 1.29 & 1.30).

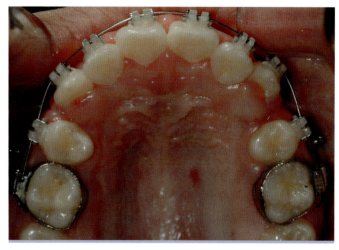

Fig. 1.27 Occlusal view after completion of canine retraction in a premolar extraction case.

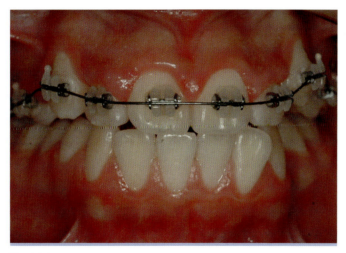

Fig. 1.28

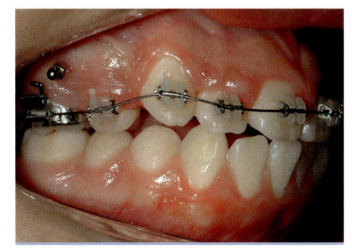

Fig. 1.29

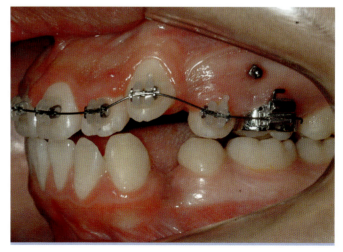

Fig. 1.30

Figs 1.28, 1.29 & 1.30 Frontal and lateral views after canine distalization.

Leveling can be performed using two archwire sequences:

• The classic sequence used with self-ligating appliances, e.g. a .016/.025 rectangular archwire or a .017/.025 classic rectangular Nitinol or superelastic archwire, finishing with a .019/.025 rectangular Nitinol or hybrid archwire (Figs 1.31, 1.32 & 1.33).

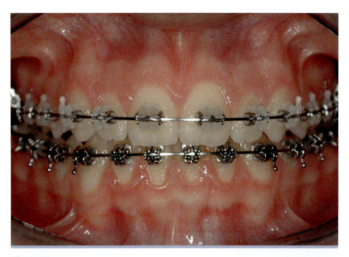

Fig. 1.31

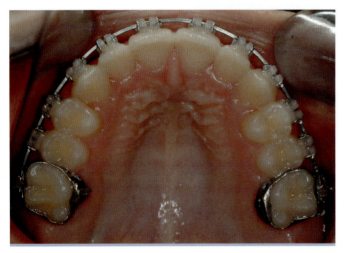

Fig. 1.32

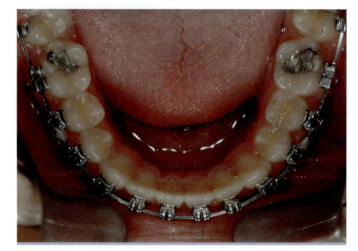

Fig. 1.33

Figs 1.31, 1.32 & 1.33 Frontal and occlusal views at the end of the leveling stage. There is a .019/.025 rectangular Nitinol archwire in both the upper and lower arches.

- An alternative sequence using smaller sized round wires that also has excellent end results and is recommended by the author. In this technique, after inserting a .014 round Nitinol archwire, a .016 round Nitinol archwire is engaged on top of the .014 round Nitinol archwire (Figs 1.34, 1.35 & 1.36). This two-wire technique enables complete slot fill-in at an early stage in treatment.

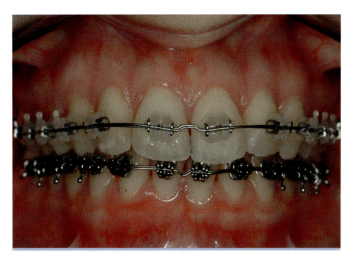

Fig. 1.34

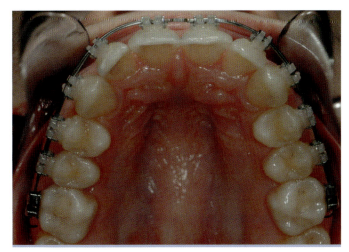

Fig. 1.35

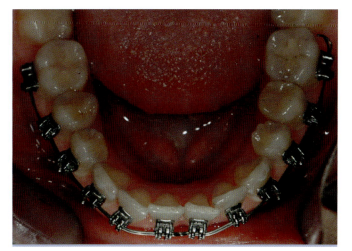

Fig. 1.36

Figs 1.34, 1.35 & 1.36 The Clarity™ SL Self-Ligating appliance with .016 and .014 round Nitinol archwires. Both archwires were engaged in the same appointment to finish the leveling.

For rotational corrections, self-ligating appliances present some disadvantages compared with conventional appliances, mainly in the lower anterior segment. This problem occurs due to the passivity of the self-ligating appliances in relation to the orthodontic archwire. However, the simultaneous use of .014 and the .016 archwires eliminates this problem. This alternative sequence is recommended for both extraction and non-extraction cases.

As mentioned above, the Clarity™ SL Self-Ligating .022/.028 bracket has a .0270 inch slot depth between the Nitinol clips and the bottom of the bracket slot for the lower incisors, and .0275 inch slot depth for the remaining teeth. This may seem as if there is not enough space to engage both wires horizontally (Fig. 1.37). However, when engaging the second wire, one wire slides cervically and the other wire slides occlusally, thereby completely filling the bracket slot both vertical and horizontally (Fig. 1.38). The .014 archwire overlying the .016 archwire in the lower anterior brackets is equivalent to a single .021 archwire (Fig. 1.39). Thus, this simultaneous use of two round archwires provides a very efficient

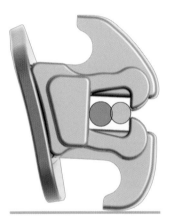

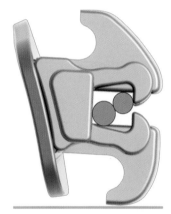

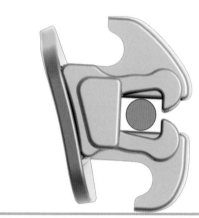

Fig. 1.37

Fig. 1.38

Fig. 1.39 A combination of .014 and a .016 round archwires is equivalent to a .021 round archwire.

Figs 1.37 & 1.38 A .014 and a .016 archwire inserted together results in a total wire diameter greater than the depth of the bracket slot. However, in practice, as shown in Figure 1.38, the force of engagement of the second wire directs one wire to the occlusal and the other to the cervical, thereby completely filling but not exceeding the bracket slot depth.

mechanism for correcting rotations, angulations and leveling of the bracket slots. Moreover, with this archwire technique, after the leveling and the alignment stages, a .019/.025 rectangular Nitinol or stainless steel archwire can be used as the next archwire. The space-closing biomechanics can therefore be applied earlier in the treatment (Figs 1.40, 1.41 & 1.42).

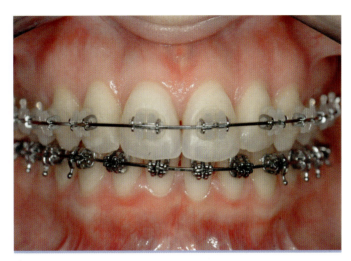

Fig. 1.40

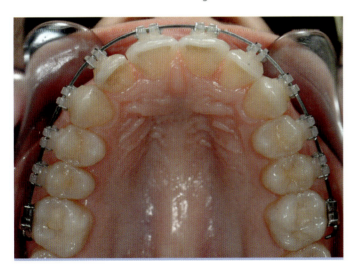

Fig. 1.41

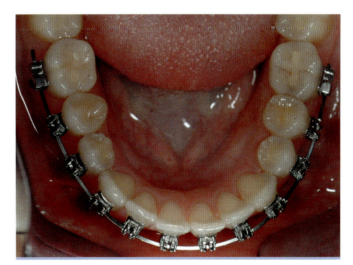

Fig. 1.42

Figs 1.40, 1.41 & 1.42 A .019/.025 rectangular Nitinol archwire in both the upper and lower arches, after completion of leveling with .014 and .016 round Nitinol archwires.

Space closure

To assist with optimal expression of the torque, .009 passive ligatures should be used from the hooks on the archwire on the mesial of the canines to the hooks on the first or second molar buccal tube along with the .019/.025 rectangular archwires. This should be done 30 days before initiating the sliding mechanics (Fig. 1.43). With the SmartClip™ Self-Ligating appliance, it is recommended that sliding mechanics should not be

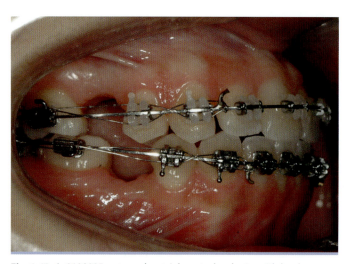

Fig. 1.43 A .019/.025 rectangular stainless steel archwire with hooks prewelded to the mesial of the canines; passive ligatures have been inserted.

used in the stages prior to the space closure stage of treatment.

After the torque has been expressed, sliding mechanics can be initiated in both extraction and non-extraction cases. Again, hooks placed on the mesial of the canine on the archwires should be used to engage the retraction system anteriorly. The hooks can be welded in the office or may be supplied prewelded to the orthodontic archwire[12,14] (Figs 1.44 & 1.45).

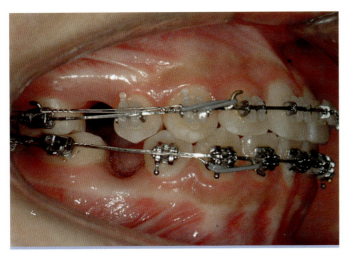

Fig. 1.44 Brass hooks soldered on the mesial of the canine on a .019/.025 rectangular stainless steel archwire. The retraction system being used consists of metal ligatures and elastic modules.

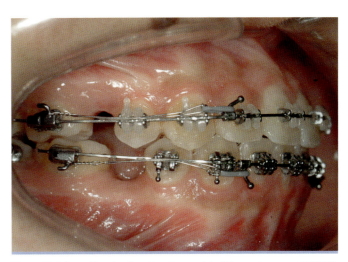

Fig. 1.45 Crimped hooks placed on the mesial of the canine on a .019/.025 rectangular stainless steel archwire. The retraction system being used consists of metal ligatures and elastic modules.

Space closing mechanics can be carried out with elastic modules and ligatures or Nitinol springs[15,16] (Figs 1.46 & 1.47). The elastic modules used with ligatures or the Nitinol coil springs should remain in place from the start to the finish of space closure and for one additional month after space closure. The aim is to ensure that the roots are positioned in accordance with the angulation and torque values built in the brackets.

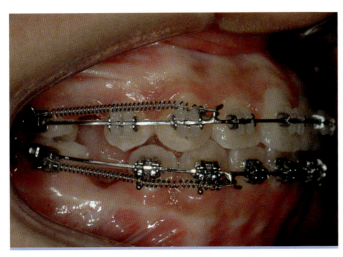

Fig. 1.46 Brass hooks soldered on the mesial of the canine on a .019/.025 rectangular stainless steel archwire. The retraction system being used consists of a Nitinol spring.

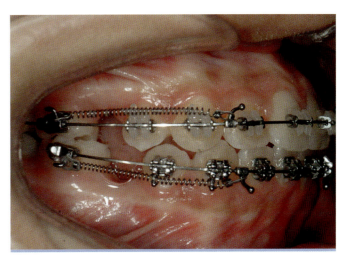

Fig. 1.47 Crimped hooks placed on the mesial of the canine on a .019/.025 rectangular stainless steel archwire. The retraction system being used consists of Nitinol spring.

Finishing and detailing

Finishing of the orthodontic treatment[5,6,17,18] with a .019/.025 rectangular stainless steel archwire is recommended after tridimensional control of each tooth has been achieved – angulation, inclination and rotation (Figs 1.5, 1.6 & 1.7). The occlusion is checked in centric relation, as well as the functional movements to check anterior guidance in protrusive excursions, and canine guidance in lateroprotrusive excursions (Figs 1.48, 1.49, 1.50, 1.51, 1.52, 1.53, 1.54, 1.55 & 1.56). At this time, a .019/.025

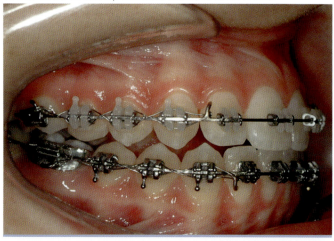

Fig. 1.48

Figs 1.48, 1.49 & 1.50 Frontal and lateral views illustrating checking the functional occlusion, that is, anterior guidance. There is good disclusion of the posterior teeth. The patient is in the final stage of treatment with .019/.025 rectangular stainless steel archwires in place.

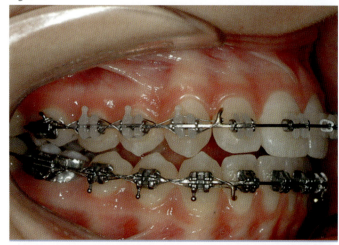

Fig. 1.51

Figs 1.51, 1.52 & 1.53 Frontal and lateral views illustrating checking the functional occlusion, that is, right canine guidance. There is good disclusion of the posterior teeth. The patient is in the final stage of treatment with .019/.025 rectangular stainless steel archwires in place.

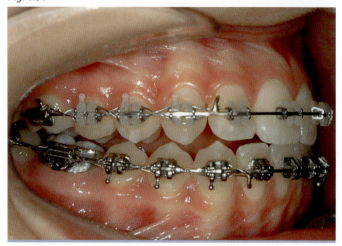

Fig. 1.54

Figs 1.54, 1.55 & 1.56 Frontal and lateral views illustrating checking the final occlusion, that is, left canine guidance. There is good disclusion of the posterior teeth. The patient is in the final stage of treatment with .019/.025 rectangular stainless steel archwires in place.

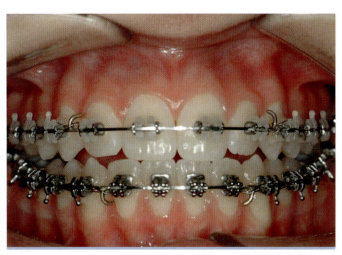

Fig. 1.49

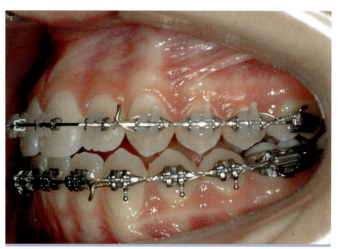

Fig. 1.50

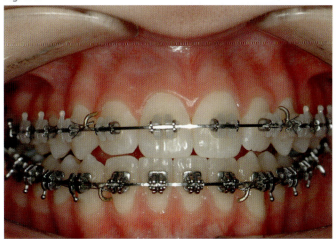

Fig. 1.52

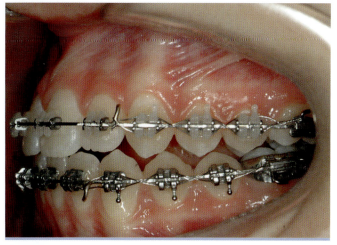

Fig. 1.53

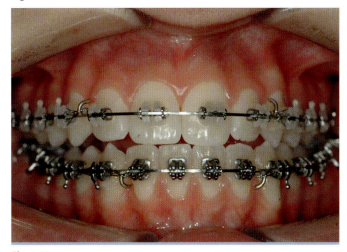

Fig. 1.55

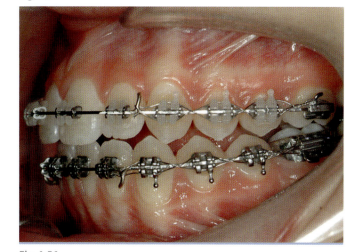

Fig. 1.56

rectangular braided archwire should be engaged to aid settling of the final occlusion, along with use of 3/16 elastics applying a 4 oz force (Figs 1.57, 1.58 & 1.59). The patient should use 'settling' elastics for a period of 30 days, 24 hours a day, and then only at night while sleeping for another 30 days. After settling of the occlusion, the treatment is finished and the appliance can be removed. Retainers should be provided as soon as possible and the patient asked to use them as planned.

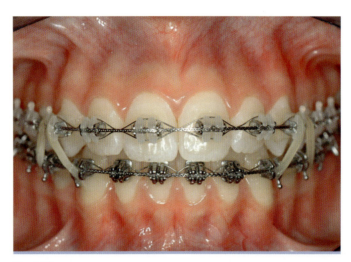

Fig. 1.57

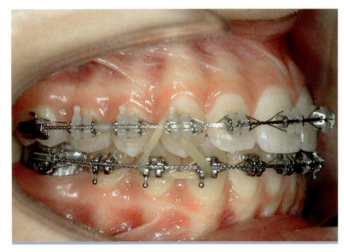

Fig. 1.58

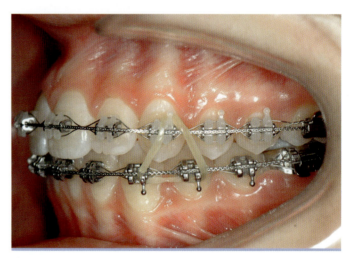

Fig. 1.59

Figs 1.57, 1.58 & 1.59 Frontal and lateral views of .019/.025 braided archwires and 3/16 elastics (4 oz) in place for settling of the occlusion.

Clarity™ SL Self-Ligating Appliance removal

Clarity™ SL Self-Ligating brackets have been carefully designed to ensure easier bracket removal, without causing discomfort to the patient. An occluso-gingival stress concentrator placed in the middle of the bracket base facilitates bracket removal (Fig. 1.60). A special pair of pliers has been designed to 'fracture' and remove the bracket (Fig. 1.61 & 1.62). These pliers distribute the applied pressure on the mesial and the distal bracket wings, which results in fracture of the bracket along the stress concentrator (Figs 1.63 & 1.64). This allows the bracket base to be debonded without discomfort to the patient or damaging the enamel.

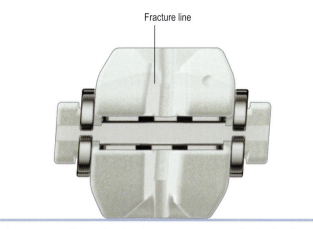

Fig. 1.60 Frontal view showing the stress concentrator line in the Clarity™ SL Self-Ligating bracket.

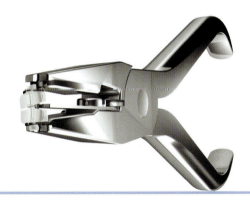

Fig. 1.61

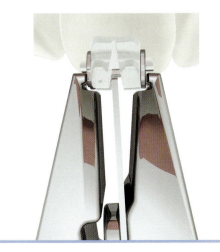

Fig. 1.62

Figs 1.61 & 1.62 Bracket removing pliers compress the mesial and the distal bracket wings towards the stress concentrator line.

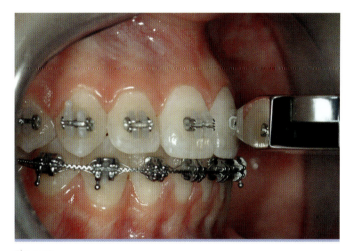

Fig. 1.63

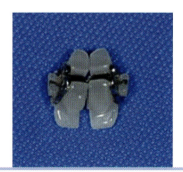

Fig. 1.64

Figs 1.63 & 1.64 Clarity™ SL bracket being removed with the bracket removing pliers. Figure 1.64 shows the bracket fractured along the line of the stress concentrator.

The appliance should be removed in two stages:[6]

- The first stage is the removal of the upper appliance followed by fitting of upper retainers (e.g. Hawley retainer).
- The second stage is usually 30 days after the removal of the upper appliance. At this stage, the lower appliance is removed.

A two-stage appliance removal is recommended because when using a bonded lower retainer, no retainers are used for the posterior segment on the mandibular arch. When the appliance is removed from both the upper and lower arches at the same visit, there may be more natural lingual inclination of the lower teeth than the upper teeth in the posterior segment. The described protocol aims at improving the settling of the natural occlusion, allowing the musculature and the masticatory function to work favorably with the functional dynamics of the occlusion, and thus controlling the lingual inclination of the lower teeth (Figs 1.65, 1.66, 1.67, 1.68, 1.69 & 1.70).

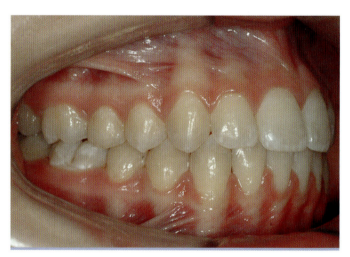

Figs 1.65, 1.66 & 1.67 Post-treatment frontal and lateral views of the upper and lower dental arches.

Fig. 1.65

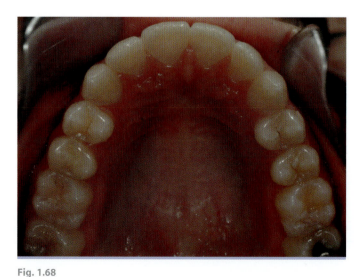

Figs 1.68, 1.69 & 1.70 Post-treatment occlusal views of the upper and lower dental arches. Anterior guidance and canine guidance (Fig. 1.70) after finishing the orthodontic treatment.

Fig. 1.68

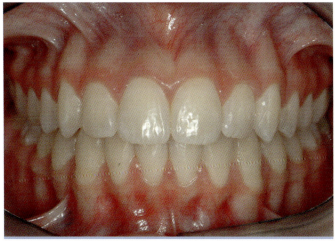

Fig. 1.66

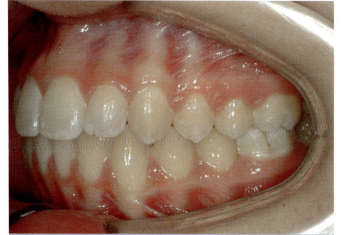

Fig. 1.67

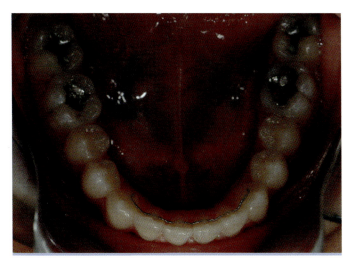

Fig. 1.69

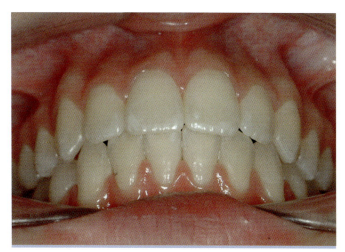

Fig. 1.70

References

1. Fernandez L, Canut J A 1999 In vitro comparison of the retention capacity of new aesthetic brackets. European Journal of Orthodontics 21:71–77

2. Johnson G, Walker M P, Kula K 2004 Fracture strength of ceramic bracket tie wings subjected to tension. Angle Orthodontist 75:95–100

3. Gottlieb E L, Nelson A H, Vogels D S, 3rd 1991 1990 JCO study of orthodontic diagnosis and treatment procedures.1. Results and trends. Journal of Clinical Orthodontics 25:145–156

4. Trevisi H 2007 SmartClip™: tratamento ortodôntico com sistema de aparelho autoligado – conceito e biomecânica. Elsevier, Rio de Janeiro

5. Bennett J C, McLaughlin R P 1998 O tratamento ortodôntico da dentição com o aparelho pré-ajustado. Artes Médicas, São Paulo, pp 28–40

6. McLaughlin R P, Bennett J C, Trevisi H 2004 Mecânica sistematizada de tratamento ortodôntico. Artes Médicas, São Paulo

7. Hawley C A 1905 Determination of the normal arch and its application to orthodontics. Dental Cosmos 47:541–552

8. McLaughlin R P, Bennett J C 1999 Arch form considerations for stability and esthetics. Revista Española de Ortodoncia 29:46–63

9. Kim T K, Kim K D, Baek S H 2008 Comparison of frictional forces during the initial leveling stage in various combinations of self-ligating brackets and archwires with a custom-designed typodont system. American Journal of Orthodontics and Dentofacial Orthopedics 133:187

10. Yeh C L, Kusnoto B, Viana G, Evans C A, Drummond J L 2007 In-vitro evaluation of frictional resistance between brackets with passive-ligation designs. American Journal of Orthodontics and Dentofacial Orthopedics 131:704

11. Kusy R P, Whitley J Q 2001 Frictional resistance of metal-lined ceramic brackets versus conventional stainless steel brackets and development of 3-D friction maps. Angle Orthodontist 71:364–374

12. Bennett J C, McLaughlin R P 1990 Controlled space closure with a preadjusted appliance system. Journal of Clinical Orthodontics 24:251–260

13. Zanelato A C T, Trevisi H, Zanelato R C T, Zanelato A C T, Trevisi R C 2006 Análise da Movimentação Dentária (VTO dentário). Revista Clínica de Ortodontia 5:59–65

14. Nattrass C, Ireland A J, Sherriff M 1998 The effect of environmental factors on elastomeric chain and nickel titanium coil springs. European Journal of Orthodontics 20:169–176

15. Samuels R H, Rudge S J, Mair L H 1993 A comparison of the rate of space closure using a nickel-titanium spring and an elastic module: a clinical study. American Journal of Orthodontics and Dentofacial Orthopedics 103:464–467

16. McLaughlin R P, Bennett J C 1991 Finishing and detailing with a preadjusted appliance system. Journal of Clinical Orthodontics 25:251–264

17. Andrews L F 1976 The Straight Wire Appliance explained and compared. Journal of Clinical Orthodontics 10:174–195

18. Maltagliati L A 2006 Bráquetes estéticos – considerações clínicas. Revista Dental Press de Ortodontia e Ortopedia Facial 5:75–81

Chapter 1 Clinical case 1

Name: AM
Sex: Female
Age: 18 years
Facial pattern: Dolichofacial
Skeletal pattern: Class II
Treatment time
Presurgical: 5 months
Postsurgical: 12 months
Total time: 17 months

Diagnosis

Class I malocclusion, anterior open bite with severe divergence between the mandibular and maxillary skeletal bases, lip incompetence and poor facial esthetics.

Orthodontic-orthognathic surgery treatment plan

The orthodontic treatment was performed in three stages:

- **Pre-surgical stage**: Decompensation, alignment and leveling of both upper and lower dental arches.
- **Surgical stage**: Bimaxillary surgery with impaction and advancement of the maxilla, and advancement and counterclockwise rotation of the mandible, advancing the chin and reducing the anterior vertical face height.
- **Post-surgical stage**: Finishing and detailing of occlusion obtained at surgery.

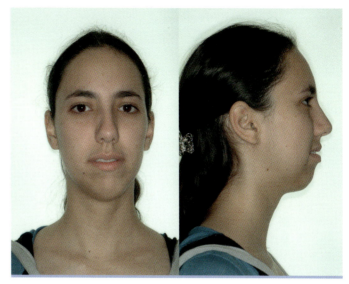

Fig. 1.71   Fig. 1.72

Figs 1.71 & 1.72
Pretreatment extraoral photographs showing facial symmetry and a severe dolichofacial Class II facial profile, with lip incompetence.

Appliance

- Clarity™ SL Self-Ligating Appliance in the upper arch
- SmartClip™ Self-Ligating Appliance in the lower arch
- Hawley retainer in the upper arch
- 3 × 3 fixed retainer in the lower arch

Case report

The patient presented with an anterior open bite with Class I molar relationship, severe divergence of the maxillary and the mandibular skeletal bases, lack of lip seal and facial esthetic concerns. The treatment consisted of placement of the Clarity™ SL Self-Ligating Appliance in the upper arch and the SmartClip™ Self-Ligating Appliance in the lower arch. Bands were placed on the upper and the lower first molars for orthodontic-orthognathic surgical treatment and MBT™ System tubes were pre-welded to the second molar bands. Initial alignment was carried out with .014 round Nitinol superelastic archwires and finished with .016 round Nitinol superelastic archwires. Leveling was performed with .017/.025 rectangular Nitinol superelastic archwires and finished with .019/.025 rectangular Nitinol archwires. The pre-surgical preparation was carried out with .019/.025 rectangular stainless steel archwires with hooks prewelded to the mesial of the canines. The upper rectangular archwire was cut into two just mesial to the canines as part of the surgical plan. In the mandible, a continuous archwire was engaged, with passive tiebacks (.009 ligature wires) from the hook on the mesial of the canine to the second molar. Cephalometric and panoramic radiographs were taken and the study models were sent to the surgeon for surgical planning.

The orthognathic surgery was planned with impaction and advancement of the maxilla with a cut between the incisors and the canines. The mandible was advanced with counterclockwise rotation. There was a reduction of the anterior height of the mandible with advancement of the menton (chin). The teeth were immobilized for 6 days with elastics and with 3/16 (4 oz) triangular elastics for 1 further month. The .019/.025 rectangular archwires were replaced by .017/.025 rectangular Nitinol archwire, with continuation of the triangular elastics. After 30 days, a .019/.025 rectangular Nitinol archwire was inserted, followed by a .019/.025 rectangular stainless steel archwire, with passive tiebacks from the hooks to the mesial of the canines to the second molars. Finishing and detailing were done with rectangular braided archwires with 3/16 (4 oz) triangular elastics used at night only. For retention, the patient was given a Hawley retainer in the upper arch, and a fixed 3 × 3 retainer on the lower arch. The Clarity™ SL Self-Ligating Appliance provided good facial esthetics during the treatment and shortened treatment time. The treatment result showed that the functional goals were achieved, along with improvement of the facial esthetics.

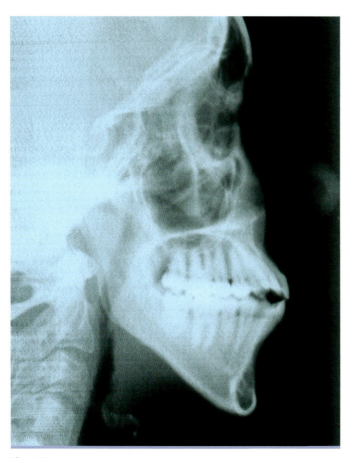

Fig. 1.73

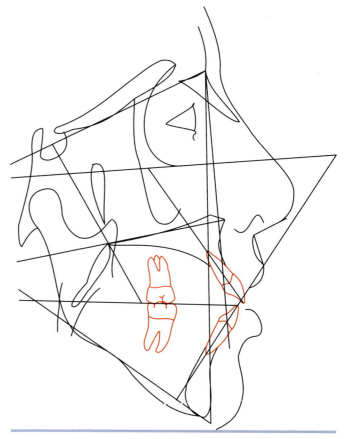

Fig. 1.74

SNA ∠	73º
SNB ∠	69º
ANB ∠	4º
A-N ⊥ FH	−1 mm
Po-N ⊥ FH	−13 mm
Wits	2 mm
GoGn SN ∠	55º
FH Md ∠	41º
Mx Md ∠	46º
U1 to A-Po	10 mm
L1 to A-Po	9 mm
U1 to Mx plane ∠	112º
L1 to Md plane ∠	89º
Facial analysis	
Nasolabial ∠	112º
NA ⊥ nose	32 mm
Lip thickness	7 mm

Figs 1.73, 1.74 & 1.75
Cephalometric radiograph, tracing and analysis showing evidence of an increase in the vertical angular measurements.

Fig. 1.75

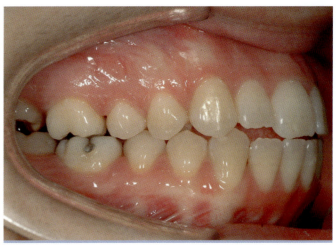

Fig. 1.76

Figs 1.76, 1.77 & 1.78
Pretreatment intraoral photographs showing the Class I molar relationship and anterior open bite.

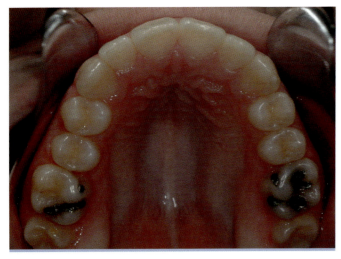

Fig. 1.79

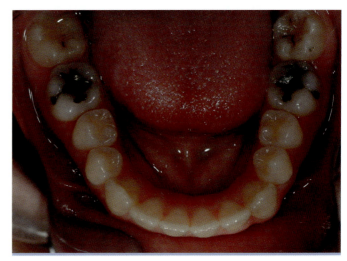

Fig. 1.80

Figs 1.79, 1.80 & 1.81
Pretreatment occlusal views showing the upper and the lower dental arches. Figure 1.81 shows the anterior open bite and lack of anterior guidance.

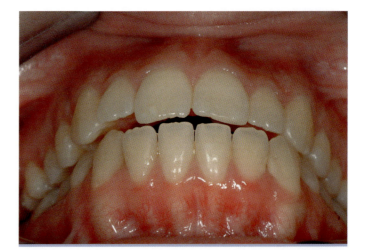

Fig. 1.81

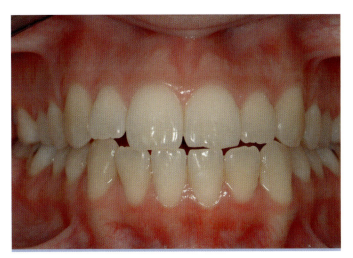

Fig. 1.77

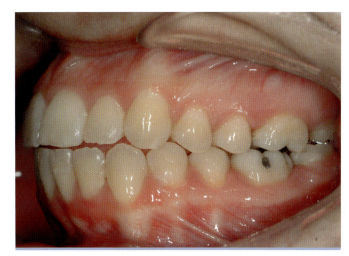

Fig. 1.78

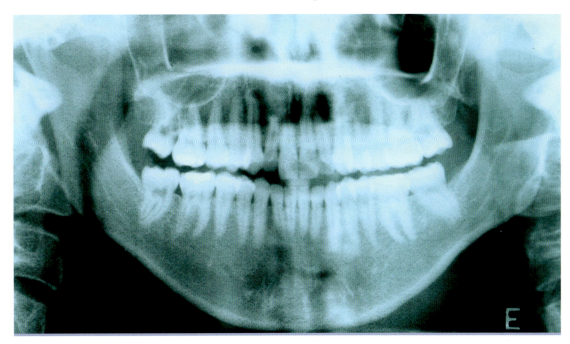

Fig. 1.82

Fig. 1.82 Panoramic radiograph showing the permanent dentition.

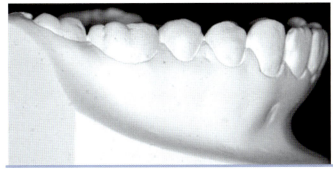

Fig. 1.83

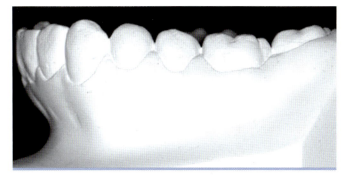

Fig. 1.84

Figs 1.83 & 1.84 Lateral view of the study models showing a completely flat curve of Spee.

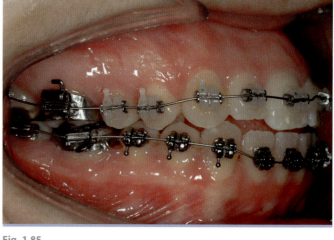

Fig. 1.85

Figs 1.85, 1.86 & 1.87
Clarity™ SL Self-Ligating Appliance in the upper arch and SmartClip™ Self-Ligating Appliance in the lower arch; .014 round Nitinol superelastic archwires have been inserted to initiate alignment.

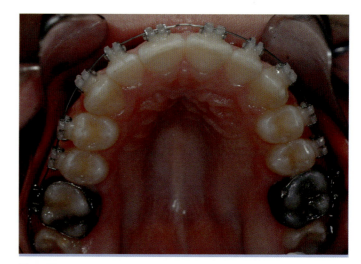

Fig. 1.88

Figs 1.88 & 1.89
Occlusal views of the .014 round Nitinol superelastic archwires for initiating the aligning stage of treatment.

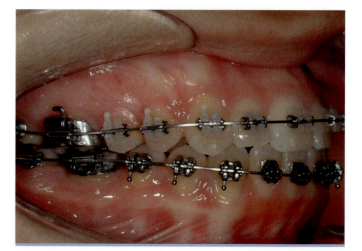

Fig. 1.90

Figs 1.90, 1.91 & 1.92
Frontal and lateral views of the leveling stage, with .019/.025 rectangular Nitinol archwires in place.

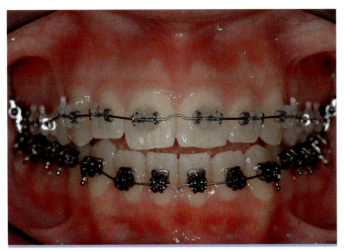

Fig. 1.86

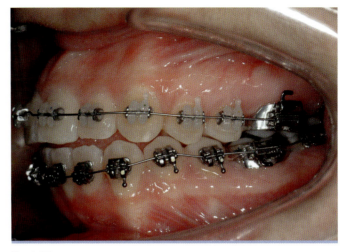

Fig. 1.87

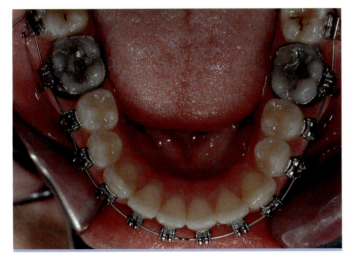

Fig. 1.89

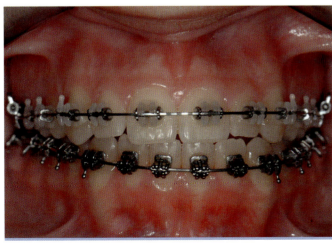

Fig. 1.91

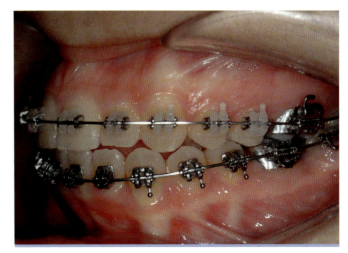

Fig. 1.92

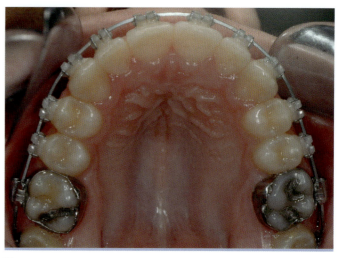

Figs 1.93 & 1.94

Occlusal views of the .019/.025 rectangular Nitinol archwires, with good rotational control of all the teeth.

Fig. 1.93

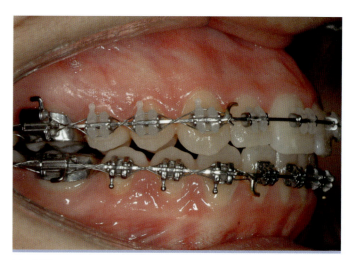

Figs 1.95, 1.96 & 1.97

End of the first stage of treatment (pre-surgical) with .019/.025 rectangular stainless steel archwires, hooks to the mesial of the canines and passive tiebacks to the second molars.

Fig. 1.95

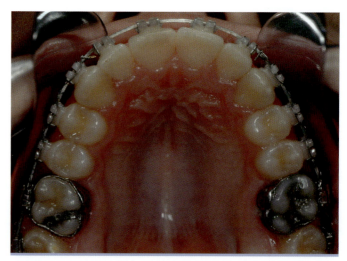

Figs 1.98, 1.99 & 1.100

Occlusal views of the .019/.025 rectangular stainless steel archwires in place. Figure 1.100 shows that the anterior and canine guidance were not achieved in this stage of treatment.

Fig. 1.98

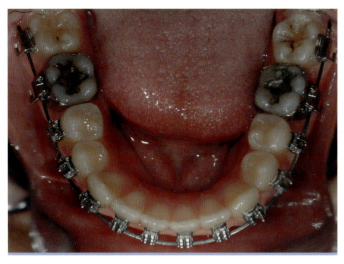

Fig. 1.94

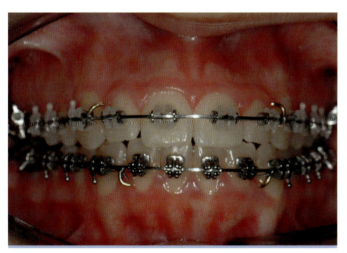

Fig. 1.96

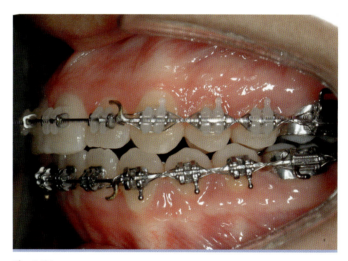

Fig. 1.97

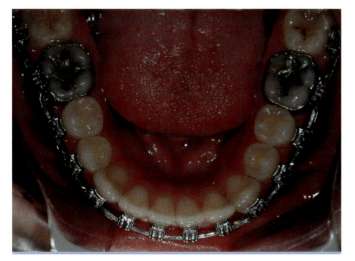

Fig. 1.99

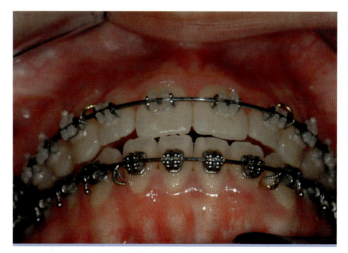

Fig. 1.100

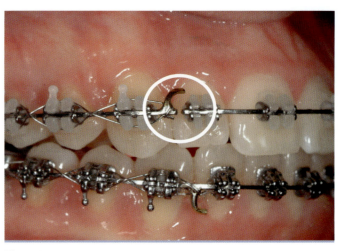

Fig. 1.101

Figs 1.101 & 1.102
Lateral views showing the upper rectangular archwire cut across just mesial to the archwire hooks on both sides, preparing the patient for the bimaxillary surgery.

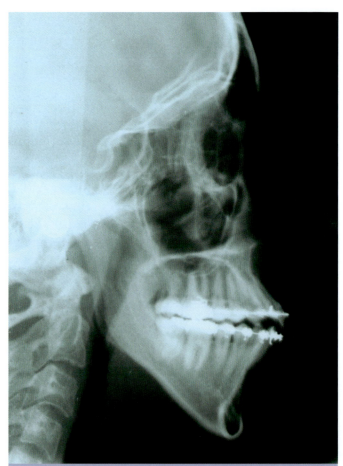

Fig. 1.103

Figs 1.103, 1.104 & 1.105
Presurgical cephalometric radiograph, tracing and analysis.

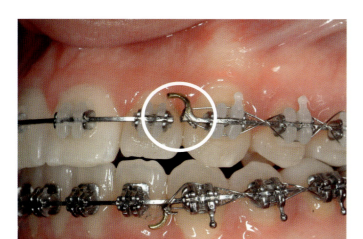

Fig. 1.102

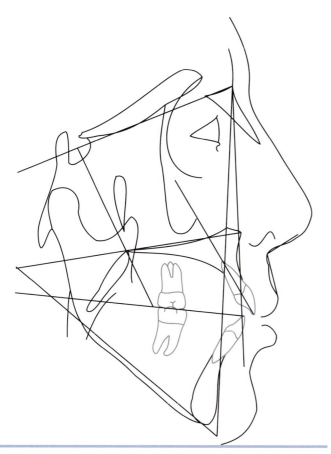

Fig. 1.104

Fig. 1.105

SNA ∠	73º
SNB ∠	69º
ANB ∠	4º
A-N ⊥ FH	−1 mm
Po-N ⊥ FH	−13 mm
Wits	2 mm
GoGn SN ∠	55º
FH Md ∠	41º
Mx Md ∠	46º
U1 to A-Po	10 mm
L1 to A-Po	9 mm
U1 to Mx plane ∠	112º
L1 to Md plane ∠	89º
Facial analysis	
Nasolabial ∠	112º
NA ⊥ nose	32 mm
Lip thickness	7 mm

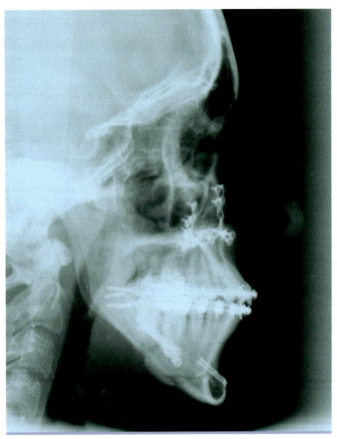

Fig. 1.106

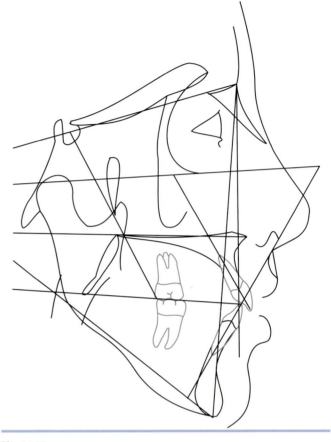

Fig. 1.107

Figs 1.106, 1.107 & 1.108

Post-orthognathic surgery cephalometric radiograph and tracing, and panoramic radiograph. The maxilla was advanced and impacted. The mandible was advanced with counterclockwise rotation. There was a reduction of the anterior vertical height of the mandible and chin advancement.

Figs 1.109, 1.110 & 1.111

Frontal and lateral intraoral views, 30 days after surgery. The postsurgical phase of treatment was initiated with .017/.025 rectangular Nitinol archwires. The patient was also asked to use intermaxillary elastics in the canine and premolar segments.

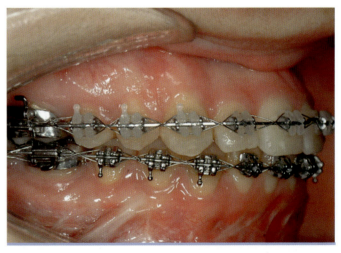

Fig. 1.109

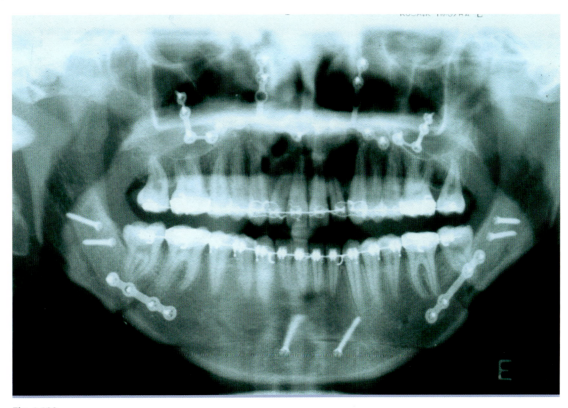

Fig. 1.108

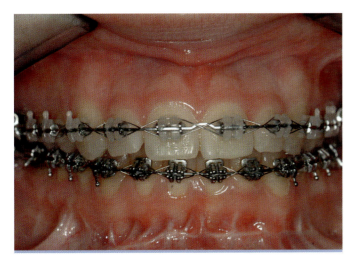

Fig. 1.110

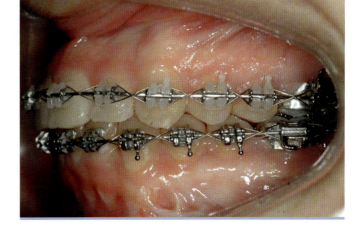

Fig. 1.111

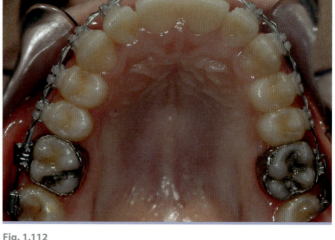

Figs 1.112, 1.113 & 1.114
Occlusal views of the upper and the lower dental arches, showing good alignment and dental arch form. Figure 1.114 shows the anterior guidance.

Fig. 1.112

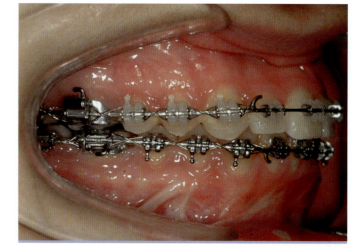

Figs 1.115, 1.116 & 1.117
Frontal and lateral views of the .019/.025 rectangular stainless steel archwires with hooks to the mesial of the canines. Note the .009 passive tiebacks from the archwire hooks to the second molars.

Fig. 1.115

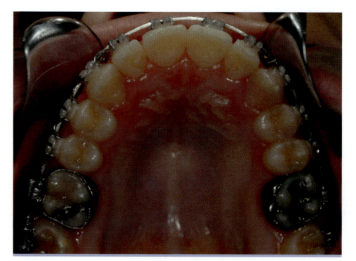

Figs 1.118 & 1.119
Occlusal views of the upper and lower dental arches with .019/.025 rectangular stainless steel archwires, showing good rotational control and dental arch form.

Fig. 1.118

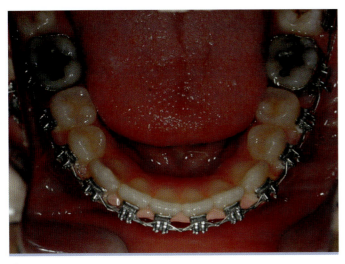

Fig. 1.113

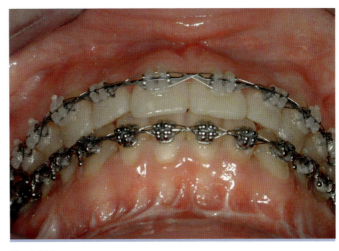

Fig. 1.114

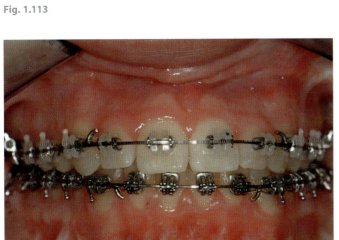

Fig. 1.116

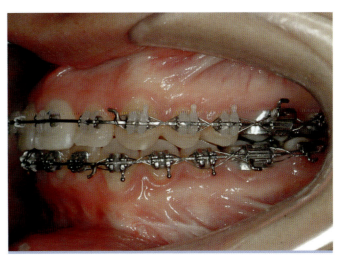

Fig. 1.117

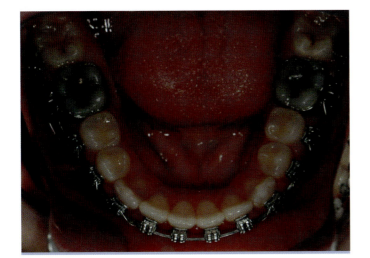

Fig. 1.119

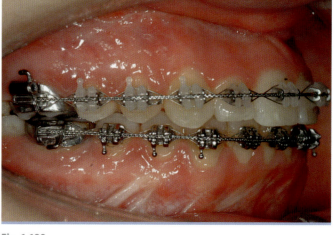

Fig. 1.120

Figs 1.120, 1.121 & 1.122
Finishing and settling of the occlusion with .019/.025 rectangular braided archwires. The second molar tubes have been removed.

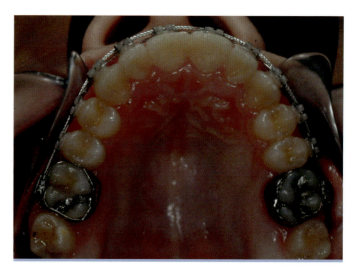

Fig. 1.123

Figs 1.123, 1.124 & 1.125
Occlusal view of the upper and the lower dental arches with a good dental arch form. Figure 1.125 shows that both the canine and the anterior guidance are well established.

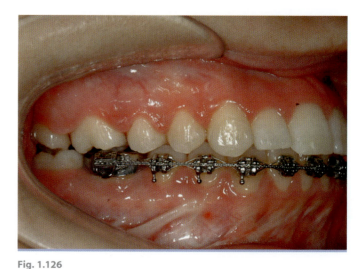

Fig. 1.126

Figs 1.126, 1.127 & 1.128
Frontal and lateral views after upper appliance removal. The lower appliance is still in place.

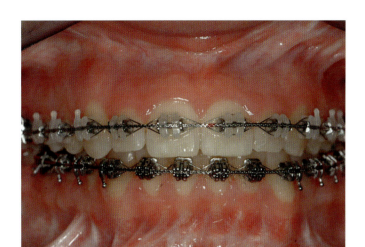

Fig. 1.121

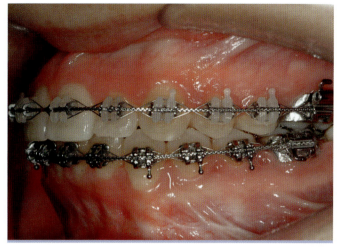

Fig. 1.122

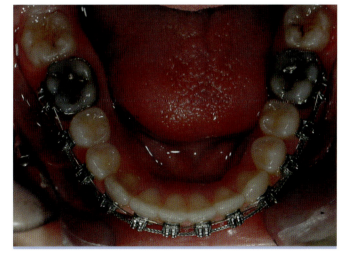

Fig. 1.124

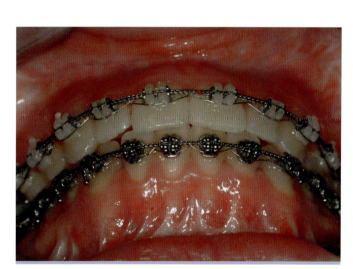

Fig. 1.125

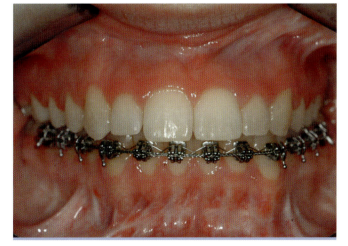

Fig. 1.127

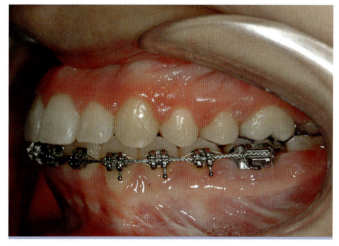

Fig. 1.128

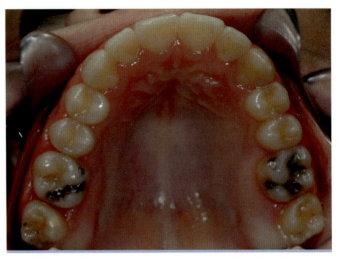

Figs 1.129 & 1.130
Occlusal views of the upper and lower dental arches after upper appliance removal.

Fig. 1.129

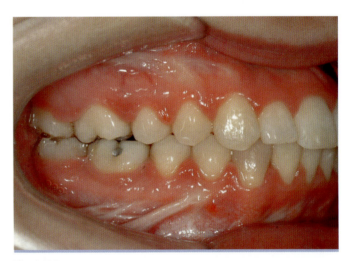

Figs 1.131, 1.132 & 1.133
End of the orthodontic treatment and removal of the lower appliance. There was very good molar, premolar and canine relationships, with the midline centered correctly.

Fig. 1.131

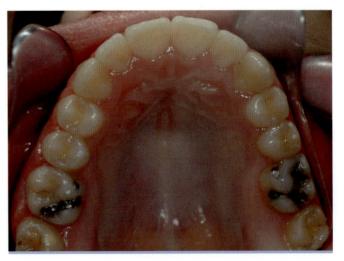

Figs 1.134, 1.135 & 1.136
Occlusal views of the upper and the lower dental arches, showing good dental arch alignment and well-established contact points. Figure 1.136 shows the canine and anterior guidance.

Fig. 1.134

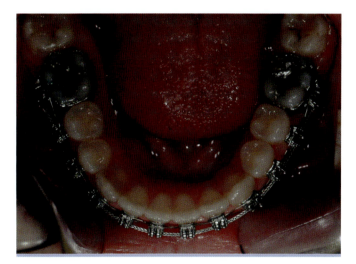

Fig. 1.130

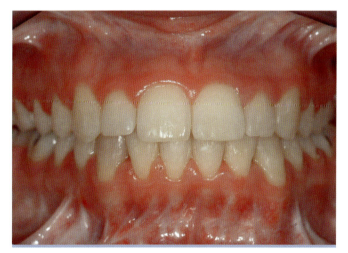

Fig. 1.132

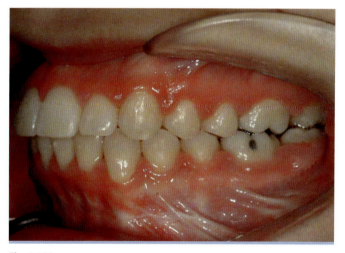

Fig. 1.133

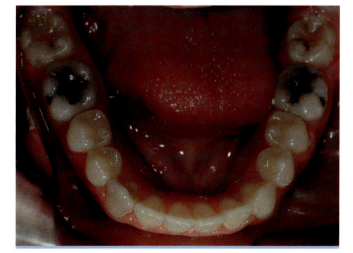

Fig. 1.135

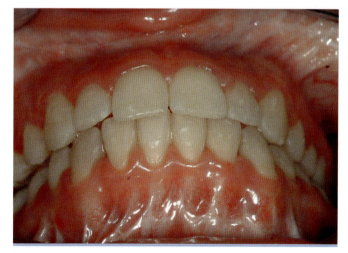

Fig. 1.136

Figs 1.137 & 1.138
Post-treatment extraoral photographs showing a pleasant facial aspect and a good lip competence. Figure 1.138 shows a good smile line.

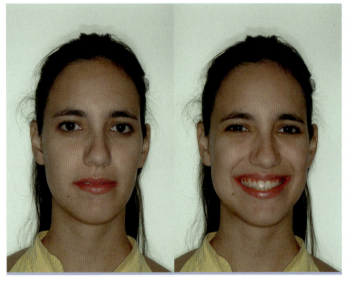

Fig. 1.137   Fig. 1.138

Fig. 1.139
The profile view showing a well-balanced face (tip of the chin, lower lip, upper lip, nasolabial angle and nose).

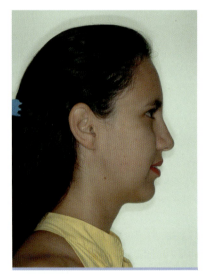

Fig. 1.139

Figs 1.140 & 1.141
45° view show good harmony of the face and a pleasant smile line.

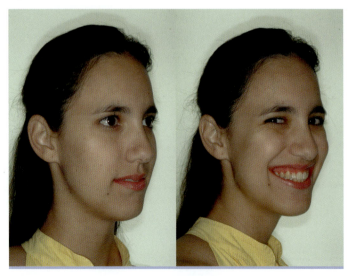

Fig. 1.140   Fig. 1.141

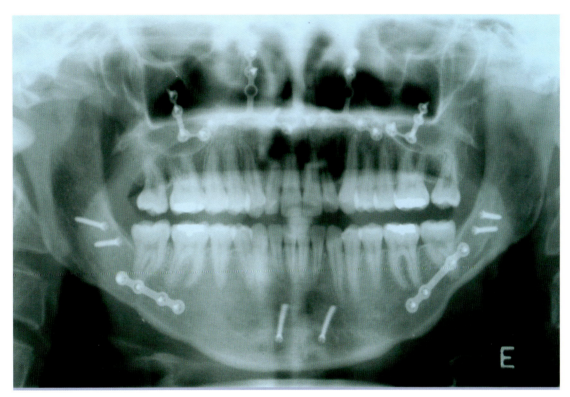

Fig. 1.142

Fig. 1.142
Panoramic radiograph at the end of treatment showing good root positions and the site of
the maxillary and the mandibular osteotomies.

Figs 1.143, 1.144, 1.145 & 1.146
Cephalometric radiograph, tracing, analysis and superposition of the initial and the final radiographs. There was a marked reduction of the vertical measurements and significant reduction of the cephalometric measurements. The orthodontic-surgical treatment was finished as planned prior to the start of treatment.

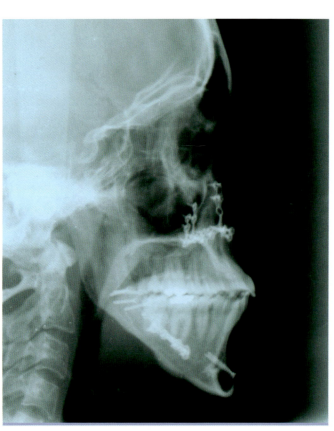

Fig. 1.143

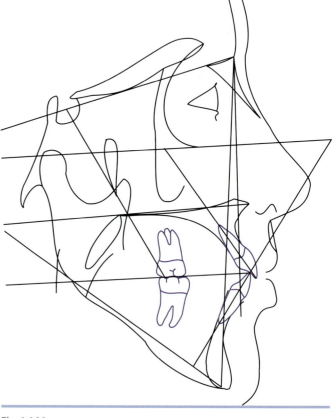

Fig. 1.144

SNA ∠	75º
SNB ∠	71º
ANB ∠	4º
A-N ⊥ FH	−1 mm
Po-N ⊥ FH	−8 mm
Wits	8 mm
GoGn SN ∠	51º
L1 Md ∠	30º
Mx Md ∠	40º
U1 to A-Po	8 mm
L1 to A-Po	6 mm
U1 to Mx plane ∠	121º
L1 to Md plane ∠	87º
Facial analysis	
Nasolabial ∠	100º
NA ⊥ nose	30 mm
Lip thickness	9 mm

Fig. 1.145

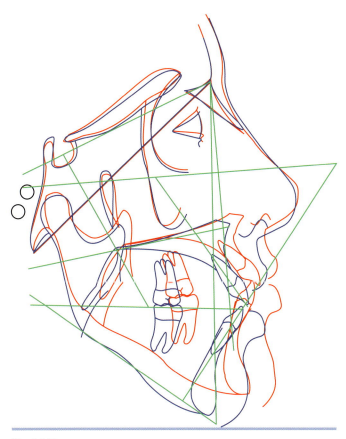

Fig. 1.146

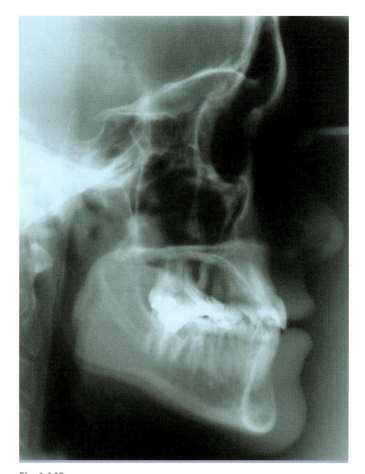

Figs 1.149, 1.150 & 1.151
Cephalometric radiograph, tracing and analysis showing the facial pattern. The lower incisors are retroclined as part of the natural dentoalveolar compensation for the skeletal Class III relationship.

Fig. 1.149

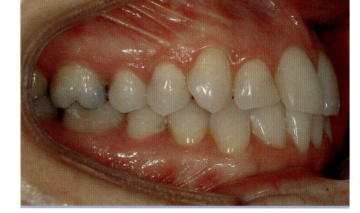

Figs 1.152, 1.153 & 1.154
Pretreatment intraoral photographs showing the Class I molar relationship with a slight overbite, rotated canines and retroclined lower anterior teeth.

Fig. 1.152

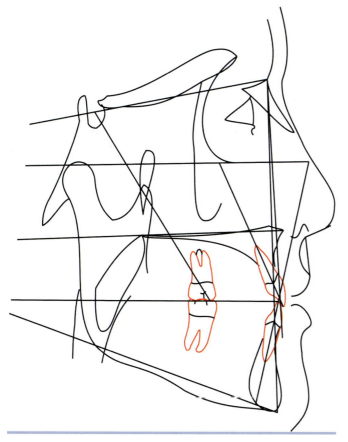

Fig. 1.150

SNA ∠	84º
SNB ∠	82.5º
ANB ∠	1.5º
A-N ⊥ FH	3.5 mm
Po-N ⊥ FH	5 mm
Wits	0 mm
GoGn SN ∠	27º
FH Md ∠	18º
Mx Md ∠	19º
U1 to A-Po	2 mm
L1 to A-Po	0 mm
U1 to Mx plane ∠	115º
L1 to Md plane ∠	86º
Facial analysis	
Nasolabial ∠	104º
NA ⊥ nose	26 mm
Lip thickness	11 mm

Fig. 1.151

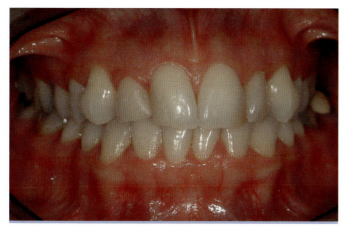

Fig. 1.153

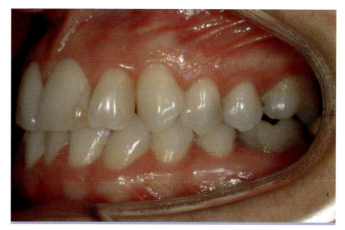

Fig. 1.154

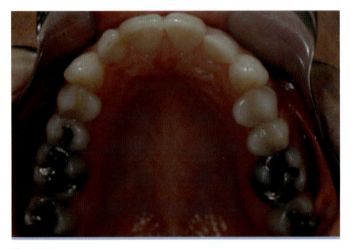

Fig. 1.155

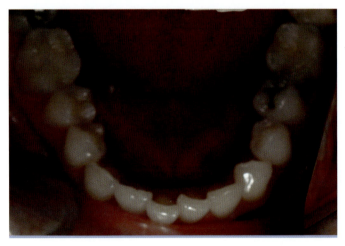

Fig. 1.156

Figs 1.155 & 1.156
Pretreatment occlusal views of the upper and the lower dental arches, showing the anterior crowding and the canine rotations.

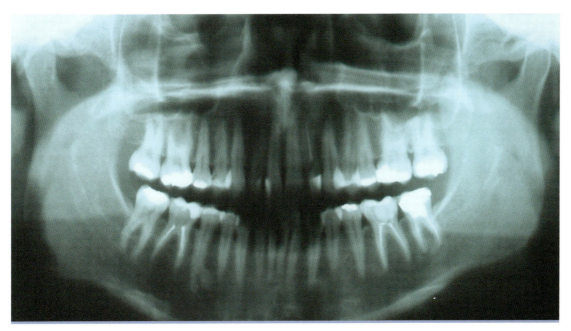

Fig. 1.157

Fig. 1.157
Panoramic radiograph showing the permanent dentition.

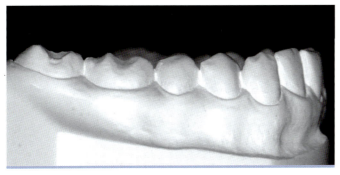

Fig. 1.158

Fig. 1.159

Figs 1.158 & 1.159
Study models showing the flat curves of Spee.

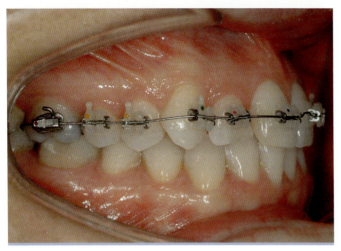

Fig. 1.160

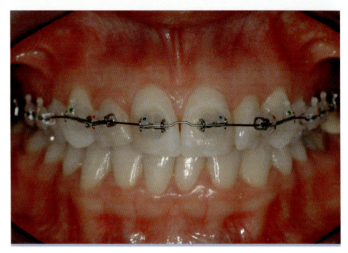

Fig. 1.161

Figs 1.160, 1.161 & 1.162 Clarity™ SL Self-Ligating Appliance placed in the upper arch with a .014 round Nitinol superelastic archwire to initiate the alignment phase.

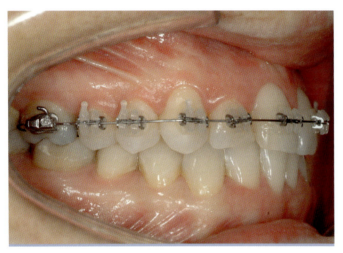

Fig. 1.164

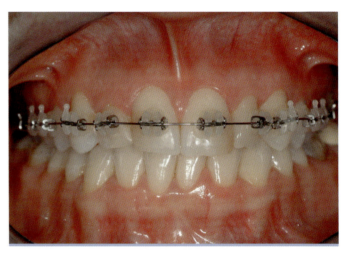

Fig. 1.165

Figs 1.164, 1.165 & 1.166 Frontal and lateral views during the alignment phase with a .016 round Nitinol superelastic archwire in place in the upper arch.

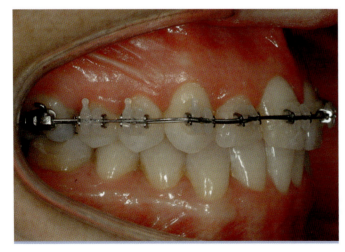

Fig. 1.168

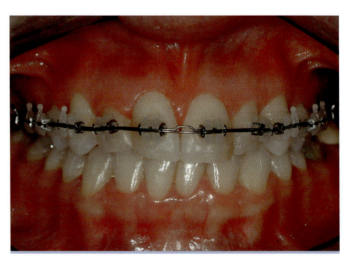

Fig. 1.169

Figs 1.168, 1.169 & 1.170 Frontal and lateral views showing the end of the alignment phase with .016 and .014 round Nitinol superelastic archwires.

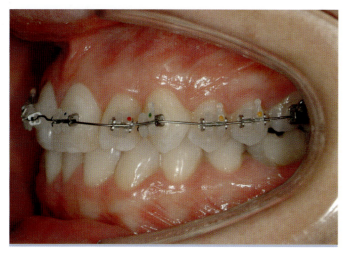

Fig. 1.162

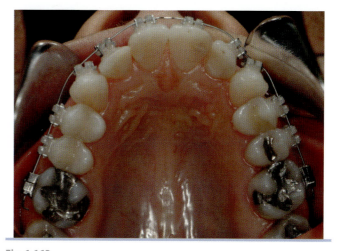

Fig. 1.163

Fig. 1.163 Occlusal view of the upper dental arch in the initial alignment phase.

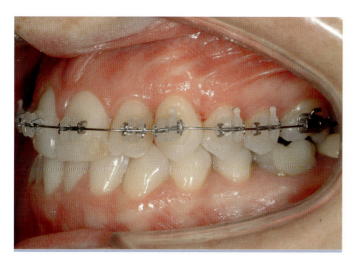

Fig. 1.166

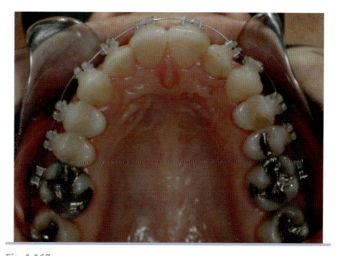

Fig. 1.167

Fig. 1.167 Occlusal view of the upper arch with a .016 round Nitinol superelastic archwire.

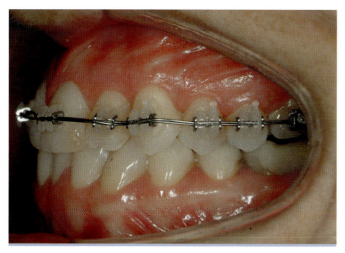

Fig. 1.170

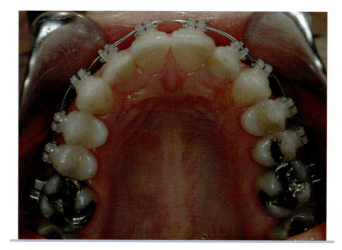

Fig. 1.171

Fig. 1.171 Occlusal view of the upper arch, at the end of the alignment phase, with .016 and .014 round Nitinol superelastic archwires still engaged.

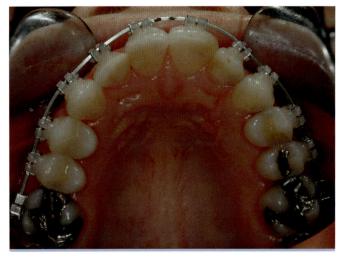

Fig. 1.172

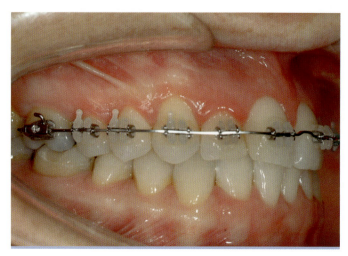

Fig. 1.173

Fig. 1.172
Occlusal view of the upper arch with a .017/.025 rectangular Nitinol superelastic archwire.

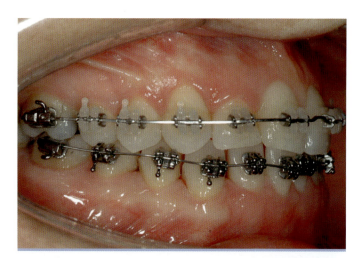

Fig. 1.176

Figs 1.176, 1.177 & 1.178
Frontal and lateral view with a .017/.025 rectangular Nitinol archwire in the upper arch. The SmartClip™ appliance has been set up in the lower arch with a .014 round Nitinol superelastic archwire.

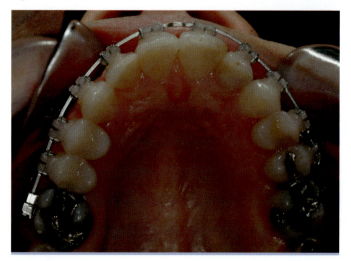

Fig. 1.179

Figs 1.179 & 1.180
Occlusal view of the upper arch at the leveling stage, with .019/.025 rectangular Nitinol archwire. Occlusal view of the lower arch with a .014 round Nitinol superelastic archwire and ligatures from molars to canines after stripping.

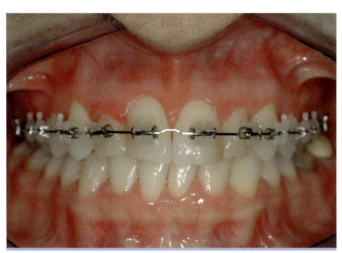

Fig. 1.174

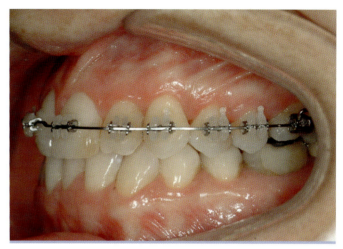

Fig. 1.175

Figs 1.173, 1.174 & 1.175
Frontal and lateral views showing the initial stage of leveling with a .017/.025 rectangular Nitinol upper archwire.

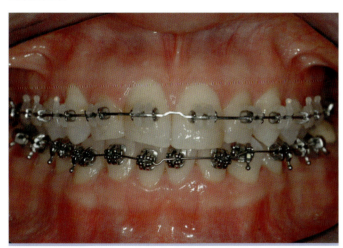

Fig. 1.177

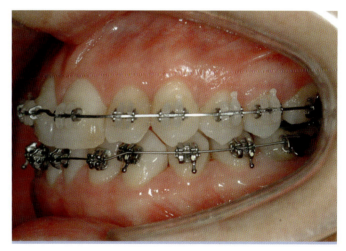

Fig. 1.178

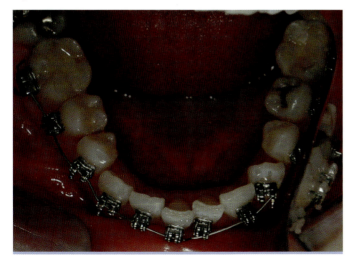

Fig. 1.180

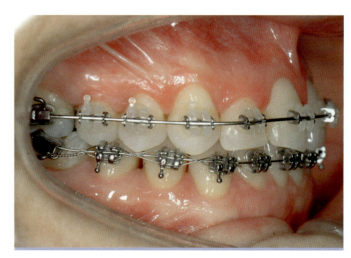

Figs 1.181, 1.182 & 1.183
Frontal and lateral views with a .019/.025 rectangular Nitinol archwire in the upper arch, a .016 round Nitinol superelastic archwire in the lower arch and ligatures from first molars to canines.

Fig. 1.181

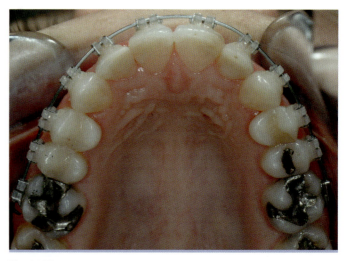

Figs 1.184 & 1.185
Occlusal views of the upper arch with a .019/.025 rectangular Nitinol archwire and a .016 round Nitinol superelastic archwire in the lower arch in the alignment stage.

Fig. 1.184

Figs 1.186, 1.187 & 1.188
Frontal and lateral view with a .019/.025 rectangular Nitinol archwire in the upper arch and a .017/.025 Nitinol superelastic archwire in the lower arch.

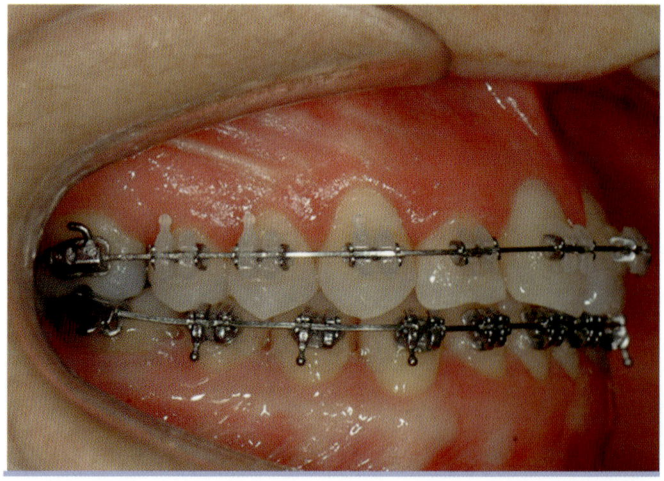

Fig. 1.186

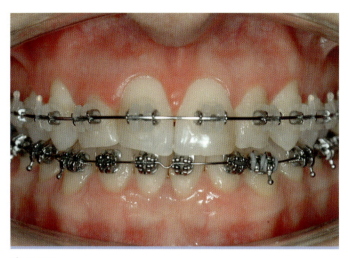

Fig. 1.182

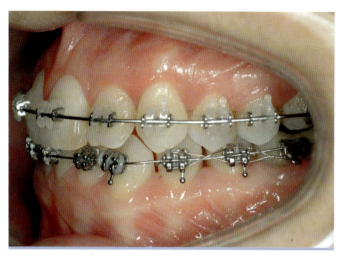

Fig. 1.183

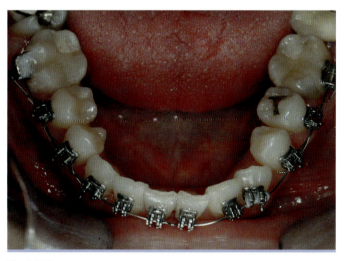

Fig. 1.185

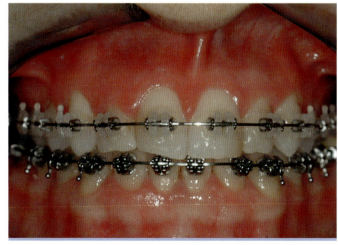

Fig. 1.187

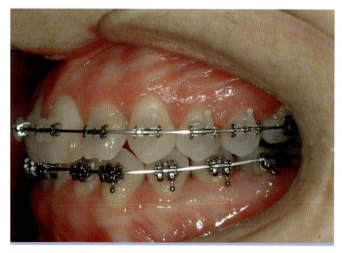

Fig. 1.188

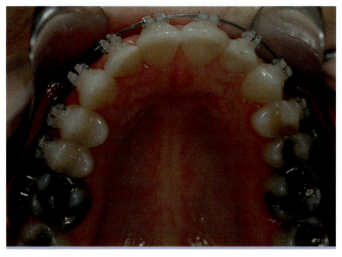

Fig. 1.189

Figs 1.189 & 1.190
Occlusal view of the upper arch with a .019/.025 rectangular Nitinol archwire. The presence of the .017/.025 Nitinol superelastic archwire in the lower arch confirms good rotational control and good dental arch form.

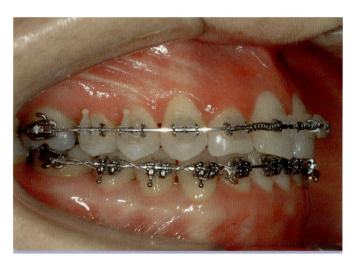

Fig. 1.191

Figs 1.191, 1.192 & 1.193
Frontal and lateral views with .019/.025 rectangular Nitinol archwire in the upper arch. Nitinol open coil springs have been inserted to open spaces for the upper anterior teeth. In the lower arch is a .017/.025 rectangular stainless steel archwire with hooks welded to the mesial of the canines to close the remaining spaces.

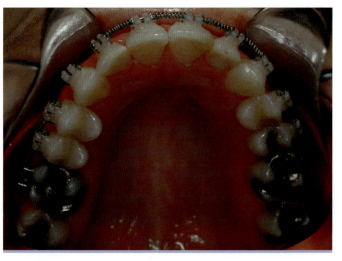

Fig. 1.194

Figs 1.194 & 1.195
Occlusal views of the upper arch with the .019/.025 rectangular Nitinol archwire and open coil springs and of the lower arch, which has a .017/.025 rectangular stainless steel archwire to close the remaining spaces.

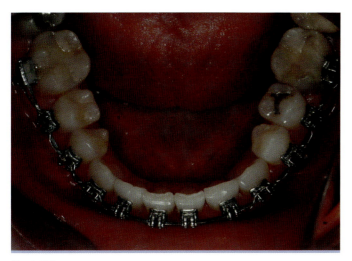

Fig. 1.190

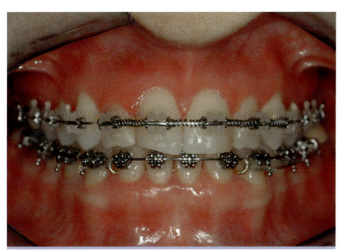

Fig. 1.192

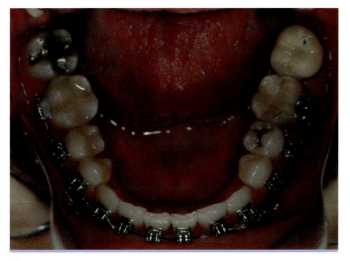

Fig. 1.195

Figs 1.196, 1.197 & 1.198
Frontal and lateral views with .019/.025 rectangular Nitinol archwire in the upper arch with spaces between the upper anterior teeth for upper tooth build-ups. In the lower arch, .014 and .016 round Nitinol archwires have been engaged simultaneously for re-leveling.

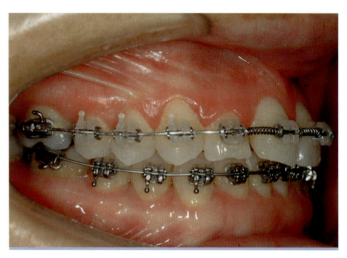
Fig. 1.196

Figs 1.199, 1.200 & 1.201
Occlusal views of the upper and the lower arches showing the contact points and the well-established dental arch forms. Releveling of the lower arch with .014 and .016 round Nitinol archwires was required due to the repositioning of the lower right premolar bracket. Figure 1.201 shows the anterior guidance with ideal overjet for anterior tooth build ups.

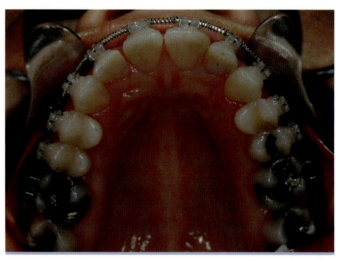
Fig. 1.199

Figs 1.202, 1.203 & 1.204
Frontal and lateral views after upper appliance removal, showing the spaces created for tooth build-ups with composite. The lower appliance and the .019/.025 archwire have been left in place and will be removed 1 month after upper appliance removal.

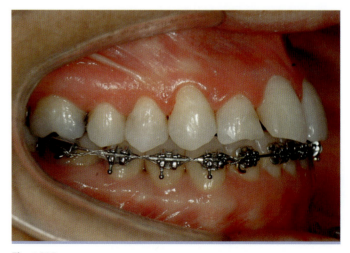
Fig. 1.202

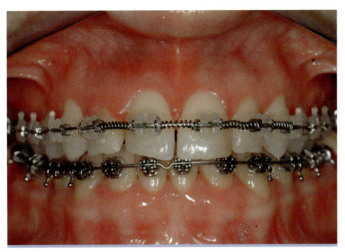

Fig. 1.197

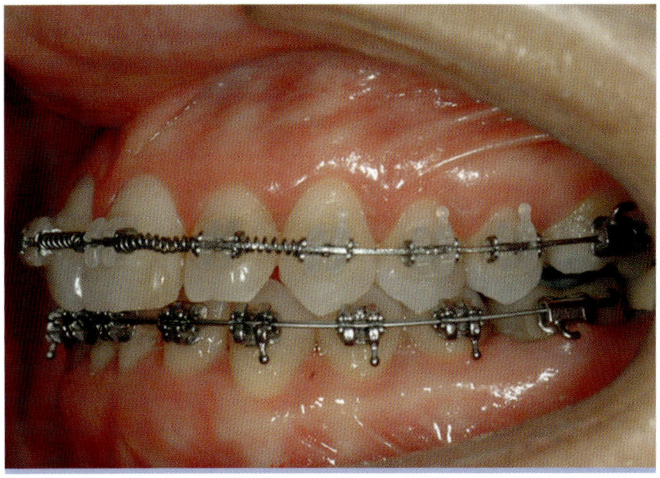

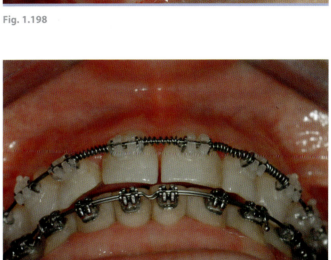

Fig. 1.198

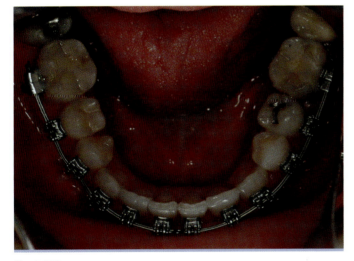

Fig. 1.200

Fig. 1.201

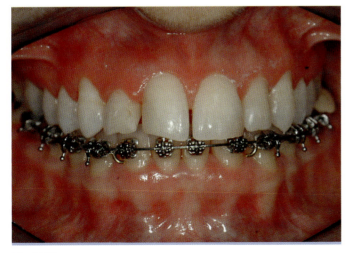

Fig. 1.203

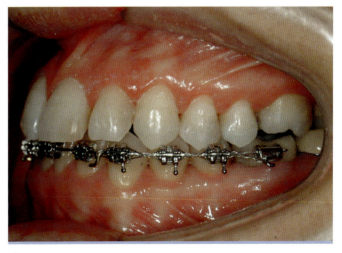

Fig. 1.204

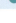

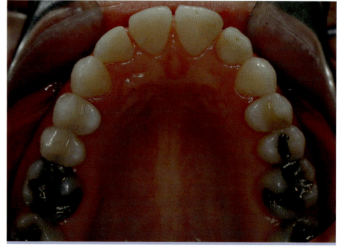

Figs 1.205, 1.206 & 1.207
Occlusal view of the upper arch showing the central incisors and the right and left laterals with spaces for tooth build-ups with composite.

Fig. 1.205

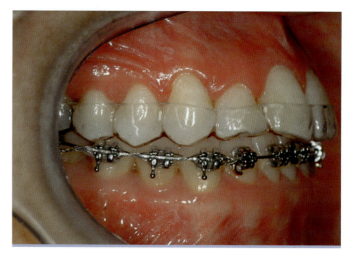

Figs 1.208, 1.209 & 1.210
Frontal and lateral views after the upper appliance removal, with a 1-mm thick silicone retainer to maintain the spaces. The patient was asked to use the retainer until the build-ups were completed.

Fig. 1.208

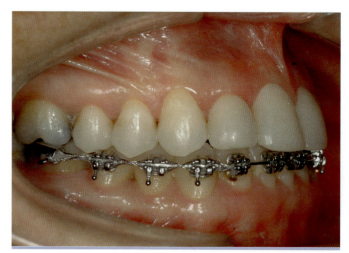

Figs 1.211, 1.212 & 1.213
Frontal and lateral views after composite build-ups of the upper anterior teeth. The patient's expectations of improved facial esthetics were achieved.

Fig. 1.211

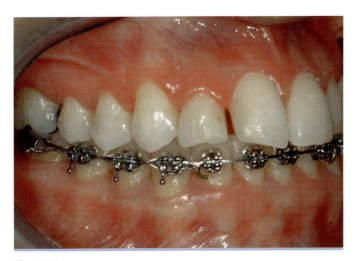

Fig. 1.206

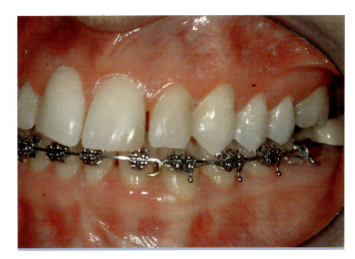

Fig. 1.207

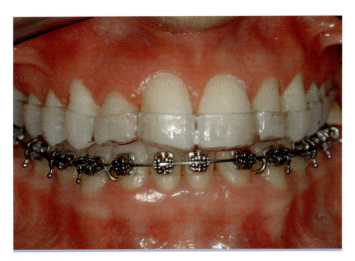

Fig. 1.209

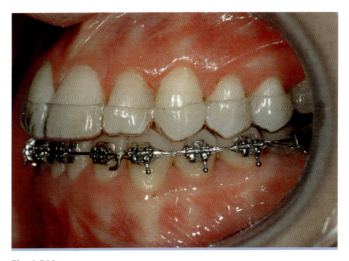

Fig. 1.210

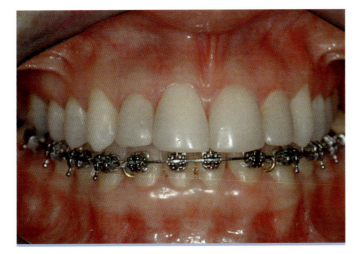

Fig. 1.212

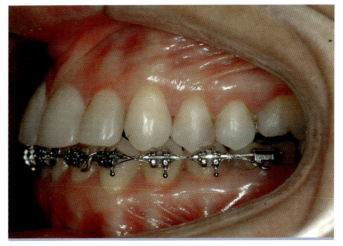

Fig. 1.213

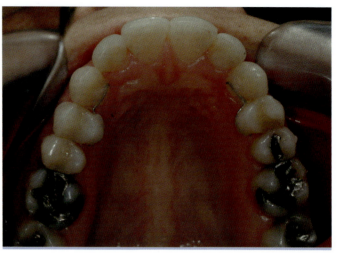

Fig. 1.214

Figs 1.214 & 1.215
Occlusal view of the upper and the lower dental arches after the removal of the upper appliance and composite build-ups on the upper anterior teeth. Two small fixed retainers were placed in the upper arch to prevent canine rotation.

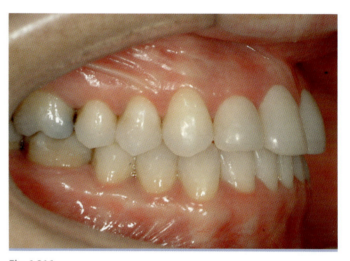

Fig. 1.216

Figs 1.216, 1.217 & 1.218
Frontal and lateral views after removal of the lower appliance showing good posterior occlusion. The canines are in a Class I relationship and the incisors show very good overbite and overjet. The treatment was finished with midline deviation due to the discrepancy in the size of the anterior teeth but without any adverse effect on the facial esthetics.

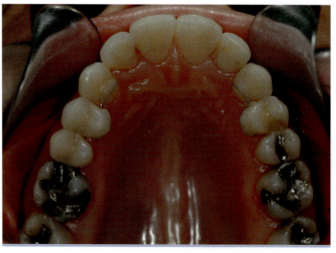

Fig. 1.219

Figs 1.219 & 1.220
Occlusal views of the upper and the lower dental arches after the removal of the lower appliance, displaying good dental arch form, alignment and contact points well established. In the upper arch, a fixed retainer was placed between the premolars and canines.

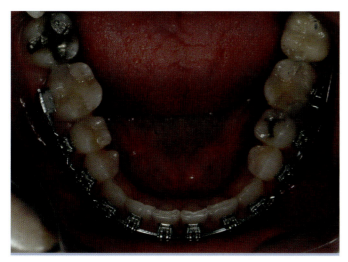

Fig. 1.215

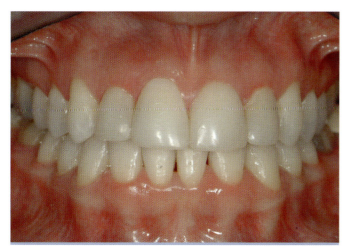

Fig. 1.217

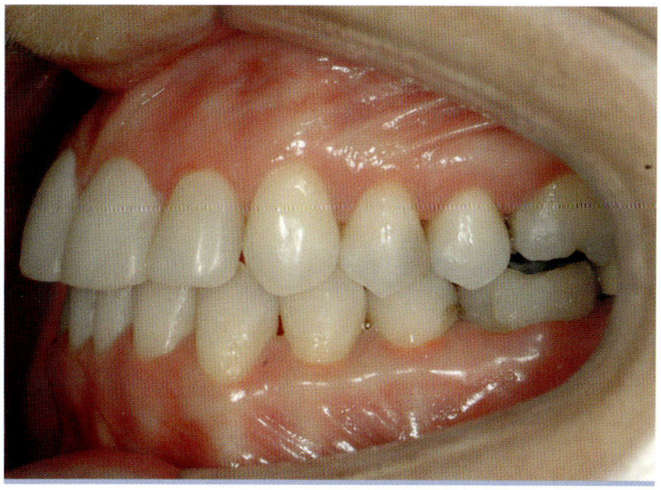

Fig. 1.218

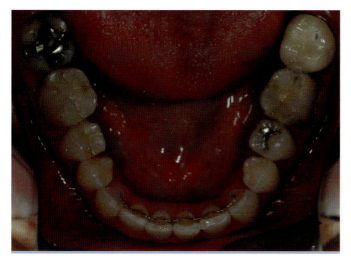

Fig. 1.220

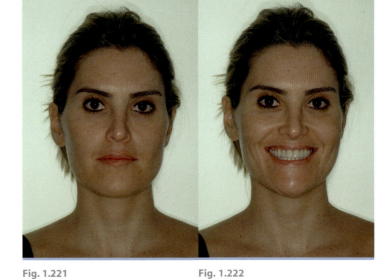

Figs 1.221 & 1.222
Frontal photographs showing good facial esthetics and lip competence, with a pleasant smile.

Fig. 1.221   Fig. 1.222

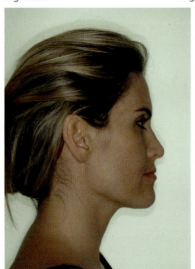

Fig. 1.223
Profile view showing good harmony of the tip of the chin, the upper and the lower lips, the nasolabial angle and tip of the nose.

Fig. 1.223

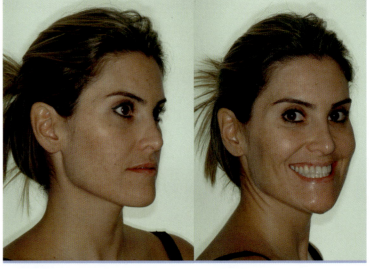

Figs 1.224 & 1.225
45° photographs showing good harmony of the face with a pleasant smile line.

Fig. 1.224   Fig. 1.225

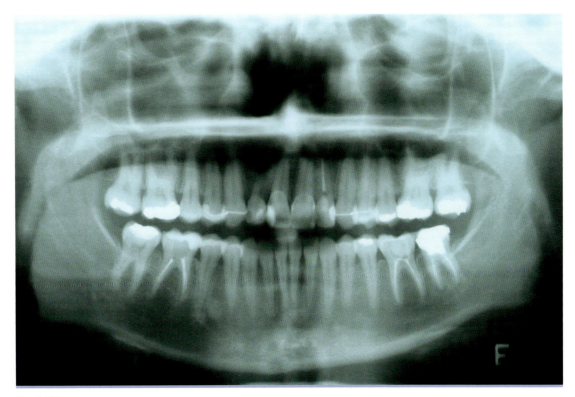

Fig. 1.226

Fig. 1.226
Panoramic radiograph at the end of treatment showing good root position. The left upper lateral incisor root shows mesial dilaceration.

Figs 1.227, 1.228, 1.229 & 1.230
Cephalometric radiograph at the end of treatment with the cephalometric tracing and analysis, showing that the lower incisors were normally inclined and the upper incisors were labially inclined. The evaluation of the cephalometric analysis was satisfactory as the patient had presented with a Class III skeletal pattern with considerable lower crowding. Figure 1.230 shows the superimposition on the SN line of the initial and the final cephalometric tracings, confirming good vertical control of treatment.

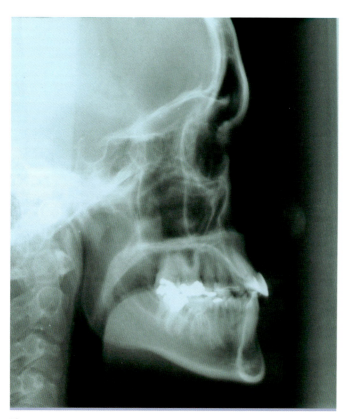

Fig. 1.227

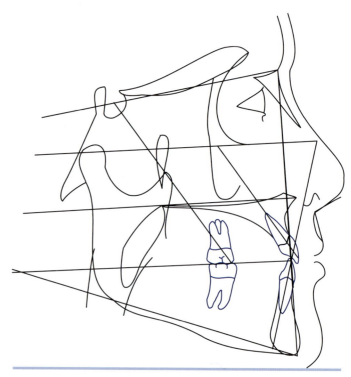

Fig. 1.228

SNA ∠	83º
SNB ∠	83º
ANB ∠	0º
A-N ⊥ FH	2 mm
Po-N ⊥ FH	5 mm
Wits	−1 mm
GoGn SN ∠	27º
FH Md ∠	19º
Mx Md ∠	20º
U1 to A-Po	3 mm
L1 to A-Po	−1 mm
U1 to Mx plane ∠	124º
L1 to Md plane ∠	86º
Facial analysis	
Nasolabial ∠	103º
NA ⊥ nose	26 mm
Lip thickness	11 mm

Fig. 1.229

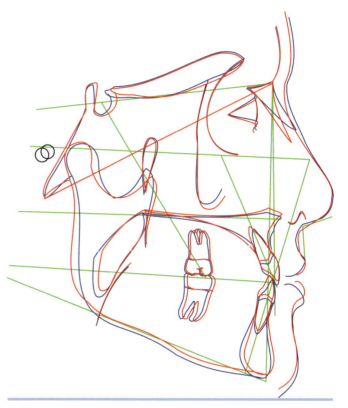

Fig. 1.230

CHAPTER 2

Miniscrews and biomechanics in orthodontics

Introduction

In the past few decades, orthodontic techniques – from the Andrews Straight-Wire™ Appliance[1] to the MBT™ Versatile+ appliance – have greatly evolved in the aspects of tipping, torque, rotation and bracket design. This evolution has been based on the search for a technique that would enable ease of appliance set up with a bracket prescription that would provide good torque, tip, rotation and anchorage control, during all the stages of orthodontic treatment.

Anchorage systems have always been an issue in orthodontic treatment, as they can be uncomfortable, unattractive and dependent on patient cooperation. Frequently, the best results are achieved in patients who show good cooperation.

Extraoral orthodontic anchorage systems include headgear and facemasks. Intraoral devices include Class II and Class III elastics, lip-bumpers and various Class II correction appliances. The most common intraoral fixed anchorage devices which do not demand patient compliance are the transpalatal bar, the lingual arch, the Nance button, the Distal Jet and the distalization pendulum devices. Intraoral anchorage devices can be uncomfortable for the patient, and can prevent good oral hygiene and sliding mechanics. Clinicians are often unable to deliver treatment efficiently or obtain the desired result when using intraoral anchorage devices.

Miniscrews have proved an excellent anchorage device for contemporary orthodontic treatment. They have several advantages including: they are not bulky; they are easy to insert and remove; they enhance vertical control; and they allow sectional orthodontic treatment in both the maxilla and in the mandible (see below). In addition, these devices are comfortable for the patient and do not require patient cooperation.

Miniscrew anchorage also helps deliver more predictable orthodontic treatment,[2] allowing optimal use of sliding mechanics with low force levels and more favorable biological responses in a variety of situations. For example: when distalizing molars in Class II treatment and Class III treatment; in retraction of the anterior teeth, in extraction as well as in non-extraction cases; for posterior vertical control in patients with high mandibular angles; and for anterior vertical control in overbite cases.

Another important application of the temporary skeletal anchorage as provided by miniscrews relates to sectional orthodontic treatments, most notably in adult patients. Miniscrews allow moving teeth in a given segment with no counter action on the teeth in the remaining segments. This is possible as the contralateral teeth or teeth in the opposing arch are not required for anchorage.

SmartClip™ Self-Ligating Appliance and orthodontic miniscrews

The use of miniscrews in conjunction with the SmartClip™ Self-Ligating Appliance[3] favors optimal application of sliding mechanics during tooth movement. The SmartClip™ Self-Ligating Appliance System with its reduced friction allows the application of low force levels compared with conventional bracket systems. It also has less anchorage requirements during alignment, leveling and space closure stages of treatment.

Classically, with the use of conventional appliance systems, friction is caused by the use of elastic and metal ligatures to keep the archwire engaged in the bracket slot. In the absence of these modalities, there is a decrease in the force levels required for the treatment, resulting in less undesired tooth movement (Figs 2.1, 2.2 & 2.3).

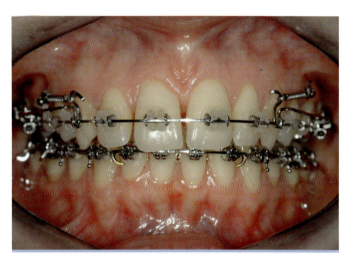

Fig. 2.1

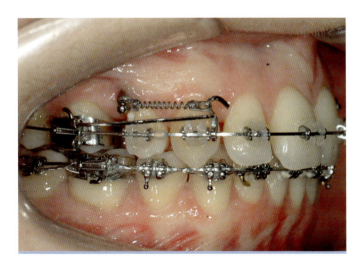

Fig. 2.2

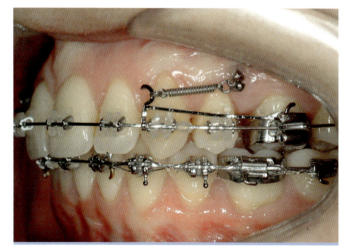

Fig. 2.3

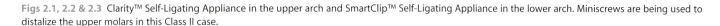

Figs 2.1, 2.2 & 2.3 Clarity™ Self-Ligating Appliance in the upper arch and SmartClip™ Self-Ligating Appliance in the lower arch. Miniscrews are being used to distalize the upper molars in this Class II case.

Another type of frictional force is generated by the biomechanics, regardless of the type of appliance used. This friction is called *binding*, and it develops between the archwire and the bracket slot. It is caused when angulation and rotation have not been fully corrected. Frequently, however, binding occurs as a result of the direction and the level of force applied during sliding mechanics. Thus, with the lower force levels used with self-ligating appliances, there is also a decrease in the binding produced during treatment.

An important point to consider when using miniscrews in conjunction with the SmartClip™ Self-Ligating Appliance is the position of the miniscrew and the direction of the force applied for alignment, leveling and space closure mechanics. As the vertical vectors are established by the clinician, the position of the miniscrews in the maxilla and in the mandible can alter the direction of the vertical vectors, favoring correction of both deep bite and open bite.

Miniscrews: type, shape and size

There are several types of orthodontic miniscrew.[4] The Unitek™ Temporary Anchorage Device (TAD) System is a self-tapping system that does not require pre-drilling of the cortical plate or the alveolar bone. The Unitek™ TAD features a 4 mm tapered body shape and, because it is a self-tapping system, its insertion is easier as there is no need for heavy force application.

The Unitek TAD System is a simple miniscrew system with three sizes of miniscrew – 6 mm, 8 mm and 10 mm – all of which have an identical shape and a diameter of 1.6 mm in the superior part of the body. Thus, once the size is selected, it can be used in any anchorage-requiring situation and in any type of malocclusion in both the maxilla and the mandible.

The other characteristics of the Unitek TAD System are (for all three sizes):

• Ball-shaped head with two perforations which is 2.4 mm in length (including the grooved neck)

• Screwdriver squared-hold fitting (1.5 mm), which enhances the ease of guiding and insertion of the device

• 1 mm transmucosal collar

• Body length of 2 mm for the 6 mm miniscrew, 4 mm length for the 8mm miniscrew and 6 mm length for the 10 mm miniscrew

• 4 mm tapered body length (Fig. 2.4).

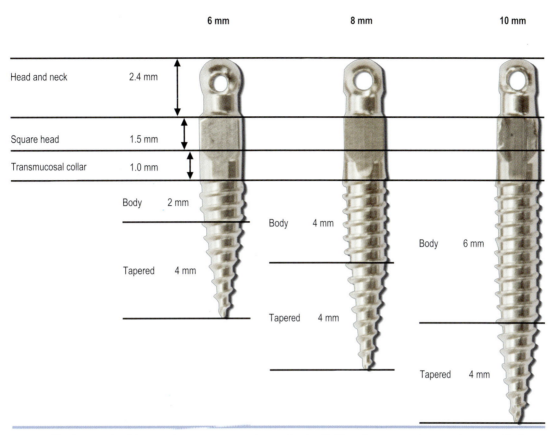

6 mm   8 mm   10 mm

Head and neck   2.4 mm

Square head   1.5 mm

Transmucosal collar   1.0 mm

Body   2 mm

Tapered   4 mm

Body   4 mm

Tapered   4 mm

Body   6 mm

Tapered   4 mm

Fig. 2.4 The three kinds of the Unitek™ Temporary Anchorage Device (TAD) Implants: 6 mm, 8 mm and 10 mm. All of them feature the same 2.4 mm head and neck; 1.5 mm square abutment; 1 mm transmucosal collar; 1.8 mm diameter body; and 4 mm tapered body.

Surgical protocol for the insertion of miniscrews

The surgical protocol[5] has three important steps that should be carefully planned. The stability of the miniscrew device in either the maxilla or the mandible depends on both proper positioning of the miniscrew and on the clinician carefully following the steps of insertion, which are as follows:

1. A periapical radiograph should be at hand to check root positioning and the amount of interradicular space available for insertion of the miniscrew (Fig. 2.5).

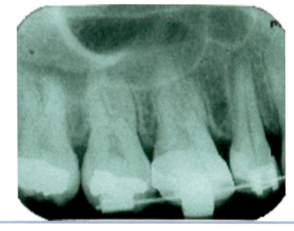

Fig. 2.5 Periapical radiograph showing the ideal place for insertion of a miniscrew between the first molar and the upper second premolar.

2. One hour before the insertion of the miniscrew, ask the patient to take acetaminophen (paracetamol).

3. Ask the patient to brush their teeth to remove plaque and any food residues. The patient should rinse after brushing, leaving no toothpaste in the mouth.

4. After the patient has brushed, check the mouth to ensure it is adequately clean. If plaque or any food debris is found, ask the patient to brush again and rinse thoroughly.

5. The patient should then rinse with 15 mL of 0.12% chlorhexidine gluconate for 30 seconds to establish an antibacterial milieu prior to and during the surgical procedure.

6. Prepare the area of the face surrounding the mouth with iodinated alcohol (Fig. 2.6).

7. Drape the sterile surgical field to prevent contamination (Fig. 2.7).

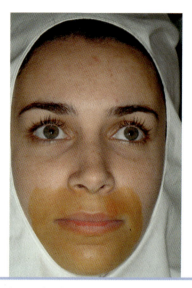

Fig. 2.7 Draping the sterilized surgical field to protect against any contamination.

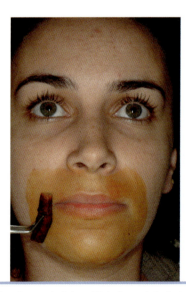

Fig. 2.6 Preparing the surgical site with iodinated alcohol.

8. Apply a topical anesthetic (lidocaine 25 mg).

9. Use infiltration anesthesia (prilocaine 3% [Citanest 3%]). The amount of infiltrative anesthetic used should be approximately 1/16 of the anesthetic cartridge, just enough to anesthetize the gingiva and the periosteum at the insertion site of the miniscrew (Fig. 2.8). This will allow insertion of the miniscrew without any pain or discomfort (if the patient complains about discomfort, it indicates contact with the periodontal ligament or the root surface). The clinician can then change the angle of insertion of the screw, preventing damage to the tooth root.

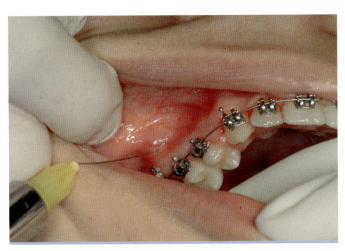

Fig. 2.8 Infiltrative anesthetic has been given, just enough to anesthetize the gingiva and the periosteum around the miniscrew insertion site.

10. Choose the miniscrew size according to its intended location in the mandible or in the maxilla.

11. Identify the site of the insertion of the miniscrew using a graduated probe (Fig. 2.9), guided by the periapical radiograph.

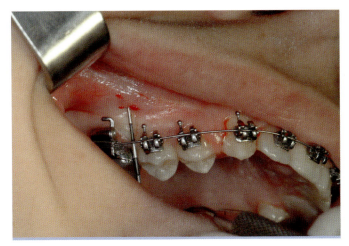

Fig. 2.9 Pinpointing the exact point of insertion of the miniscrew using a probe and the periapical radiograph.

12. Make a punch incision in the keratinized gingiva with a gingival punch. This step is optional (Figs 2.10 & 2.11).

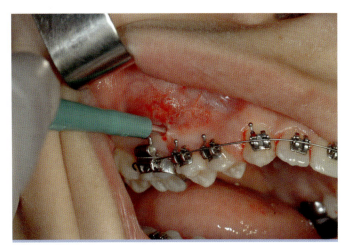

Fig. 2.10

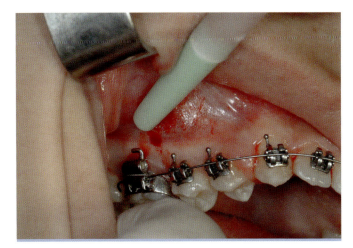

Fig. 2.11

Figs 2.10 & 2.11 Punch incision of the keratinized gingiva using a gingival punch.

13. If the cortical plate is thick it may be advisable to make a small notch in the bone with round bur or drill (Fig. 2.12).

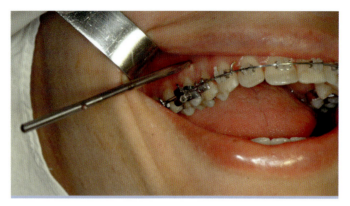

Fig. 2.12 Perforation of the cortical bone with a manual driver with no prior incision of the keratinized gingiva.

14. Open the blister containing the screw and hold the miniscrew with pliers and insert it. The insertion of the miniscrew should preferably be done using pliers, carefully checking the direction of insertion. The hands should be kept steady, and rotational movement applied with no change in the insertion path. In the maxilla, the miniscrew should be inserted perpendicular to the alveolar bone or at an angle of approximately 80° to the occlusal plane (Figs 2.13, 2.14 & 2.15).

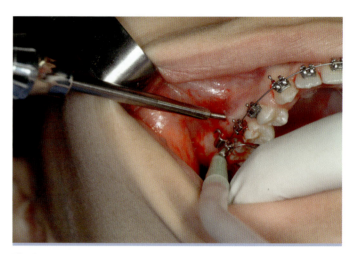

Fig. 2.14

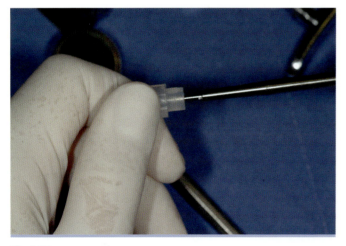

Fig. 2.13

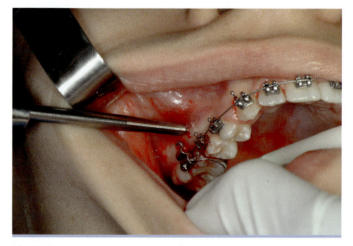

Fig. 2.15

Figs 2.13, 2.14 & 2.15 Insertion of the miniscrew with a manual driver. The insertion procedure should carefully place the miniscrew in a central position between the molar and the second premolar.

15. Check the stability of the miniscrew with a probe. It should be firm, that is, with no signs of mobility (Fig. 2.16).

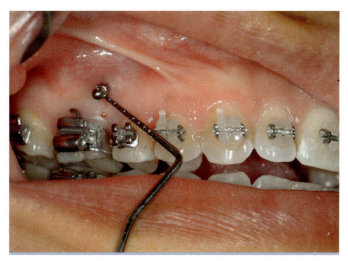

Fig. 2.16 Checking the stability of the miniscrew using a probe.

16. Take a periapical radiograph after insertion to confirm the miniscrew position (Fig. 2.17).

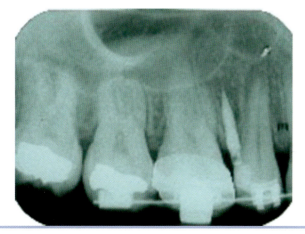

Fig. 2.17 Periapical radiograph taken after the insertion of the miniscrew to confirm correct location.

17. Apply a load immediately using springs or elastics, not exceeding 150 g of force (Fig. 2.18). After 20 days the optimal force for the desired biomechanics can be applied.

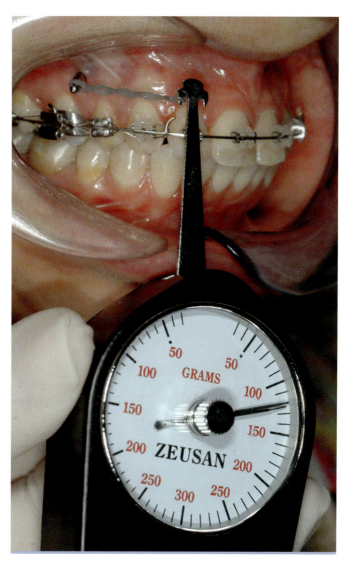

Fig. 2.18 Immediate loading with elastomeric chain. This load should not exceed 150 g.

18. Appropriate information should be provided to the patient regarding postsurgical hygiene at the implanting site to prevent inflammation, which could compromise the stability of the miniscrew. In the first 2 weeks, the patient should clean the area in which the miniscrew has been inserted with an extra-soft toothbrush soaked in 0.12% chlorhexidine gluconate for 30 seconds, twice a day. From the third week onward, buccal hygiene should be maintained by brushing the area with a toothpaste and soft toothbrush, and use of 0.03% triclosan antiseptic gel for 30 seconds, three times a day, during the treatment time.

Planning the placement of the orthodontic appliances to allow insertion of miniscrews

Regardless of the presenting malocclusion and the biomechanics to be applied, every orthodontic case requires pretreatment planning as to placement of the appliance. This is also the case when miniscrews are inserted as the anchorage device.[6] Planning the appliance set-up allows the use of well-established biomechanics with more efficiency, avoiding undesired tooth movement and decreasing treatment time. Thus the clinician should place an orthodontic appliance with due consideration of the biomechanics to be applied and keeping in mind the following four points:

- For distalizing molars, buccal tubes with an auxiliary tube toward the gingival should be used to allow use of a distalizing jig (Figs 2.19, 2.20 & 2.21).
- In adult patients, fully erupted second molars should be part of appliance set-up, with the tubes accurately placed (Figs 2.19, 2.20 & 2.21).

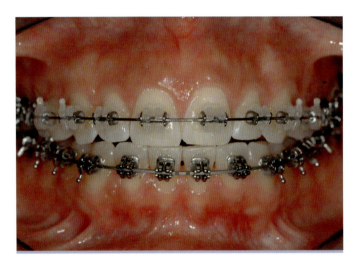

Fig. 2.19

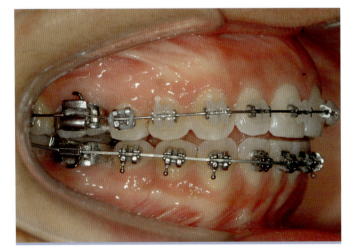

Fig. 2.20

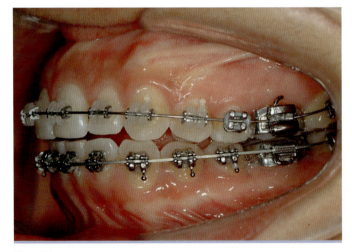

Fig. 2.21

Figs 2.19, 2.20 & 2.21 The appliance set-up is carefully planned for distalization of the molars. In this case, bands with tubes have been placed on the first molars and bonded tubes on the second molars.

- If necessary, space should be created with springs for the insertion of the miniscrew (Fig. 2.22) or alternatively the brackets on the second premolars can be placed to allow counter-angulation, that is mesial tipping of the root, thus creating a safe site for the temporary anchorage device (Figs 2.23 and 2.24). Second molar tubes should also be placed to allow counter-angulation of those teeth, that is, to allow distal root movement (Fig. 2.25).

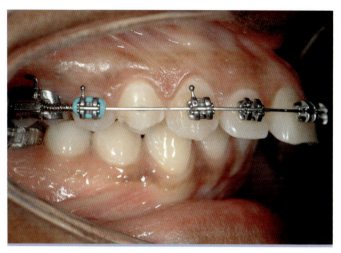

Fig. 2.22 A compressed spring placed between the molar and the second premolar for creating space for inserting a miniscrew.

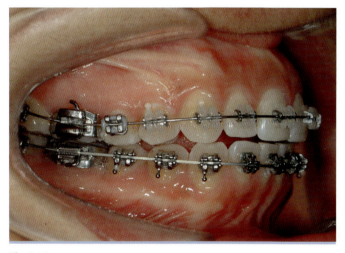

Fig. 2.23

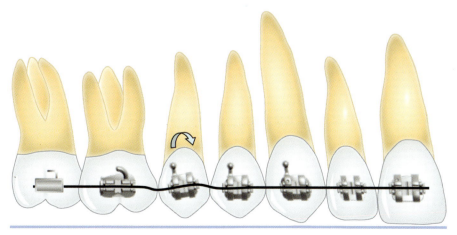

Fig. 2.24

Figs 2.23 & 2.24 Second premolar bracket placed in a tipped position to create space for the insertion of a miniscrew.

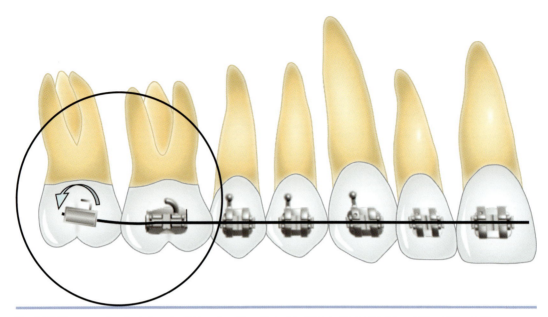

Fig. 2.25 The second molar tubes should be placed in a tipped position to favor distal angulation of the roots.

Miniscrews as anchorage system in premolar extraction cases

In conventional treatment, in the beginning of the alignment phase, when the canines are individually retracted, and in the space closure stage, when closing the remaining spaces, .019/.025 rectangular stainless steel archwires with prewelded hooks to the mesial of the canines should be used (Figs 2.26, 2.27 & 2.28). The line of action of the force applied with conventional sliding mechanics in extraction cases lies close to the bracket slot and parallel to the orthodontic archwire. To correct open bites and deep bites, bends are added to the archwire and, occasionally, an anchorage system is used.

In orthodontics, use of the dental visual treatment objective (dental VTO)[7] analysis during treatment planning is particularly helpful in establishing the precise anchorage requirements for treatment in Class II cases. The dental VTO allows the clinician to provide more efficient and accurate treatment as it enables the simulation of the proposed anterior and the posterior tooth movements (Fig. 2.29) and cephalometric prediction of the final positioning of the incisors and the occlusion of the molars and premolars.

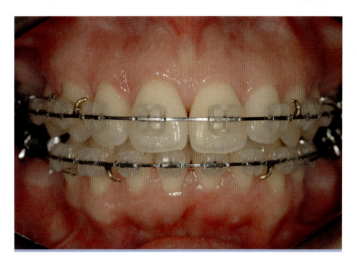

Fig. 2.26

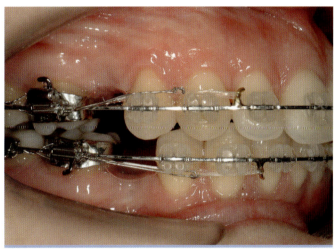

Fig. 2.27

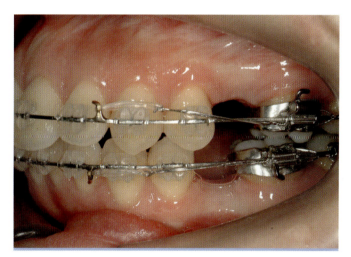

Fig. 2.28

Figs 2.26, 2.27 and 2.28 The space closure procedure using conventional sliding mechanics is applied close to the bracket slot, with the line of force action parallel to the orthodontic archwire.

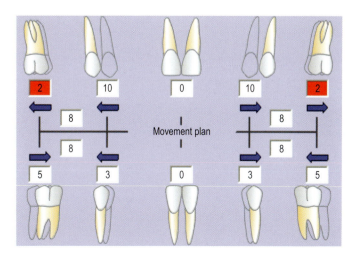

Fig. 2.29 The use of the dental VTO to plan the orthodontic treatment is helpful in predicting anchorage requirements and dental movement.

Temporary skeletal anchorage devices, e.g. miniscrews, offer the orthodontist a new approach to orthodontic biomechanics. In premolar extraction cases, miniscrews are generally inserted mesial to the first molars to aid in the application of direct space-closing forces. The vertical positioning varies depending on the vertical growth pattern of the patient. In cases with severe overbite, the position of the miniscrew should be above the center of resistance of the upper molars, enabling intrusion of the upper anterior teeth via the vertical component of force thus established (Figs 2.30, 2.31 & 2.32). In cases of

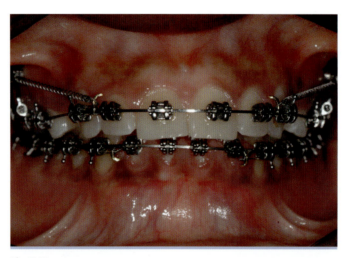

Fig. 2.30

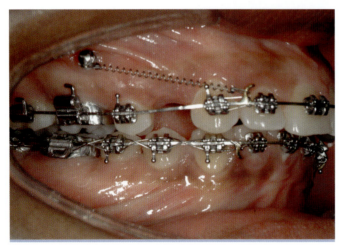

Fig. 2.31

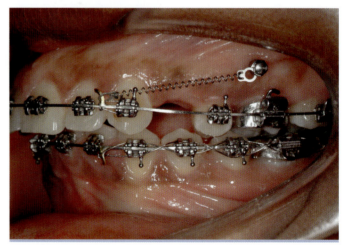

Fig. 2.32

Figs 2.30, 2.31 & 2.32 In cases with severe deep overbite, the miniscrew is inserted above the center of resistance of the teeth to favor overbite correction.

moderate overbite, the vertical positioning of the miniscrew should be in the keratinized gingiva, close to the center of resistance of the teeth (Figs 2.33, 2.34 & 2.35).

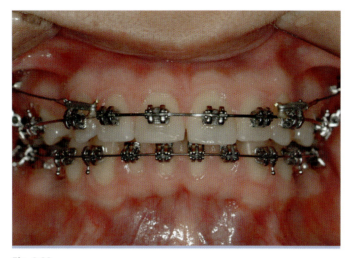

Fig. 2.33

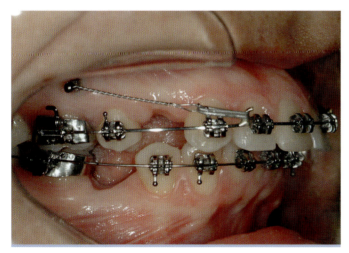

Fig. 2.34

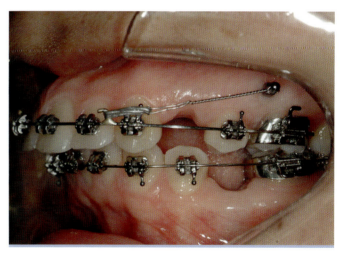

Fig. 2.35

Figs 2.33, 2.34 & 2.35 In cases of moderate overbite, the miniscrew should be positioned in the keratinized gingiva, close to the center of resistance of the teeth.

The choice of the ideal insertion point[8] for the miniscrew in the maxilla is very important for the stability of the miniscrew and the biomechanics. In premolar extraction cases, the ideal vertical position of the miniscrew is close to the center of resistance of the teeth, approximately 8 mm above the orthodontic archwire. In this way, when the point of force application is at a distance from the orthodontic archwire, vertical force vectors are generated that help in reduction of deep overbite (Fig. 2.36).

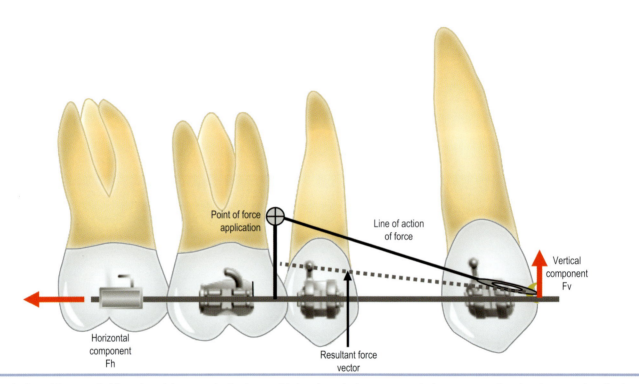

Fig. 2.36 The line of force applied from the miniscrew to the hook prewelded to the archwire creates vertical components, favoring the correction of a deep overbite.

In cases with reduced or normal overbite, the orthodontic treatment should be initiated with individual retraction of the canines, and application of horizontal forces without any vertical force components, which are not helpful in these patients (Figs 2.37, 2.38 & 2.39). After the initial correction of

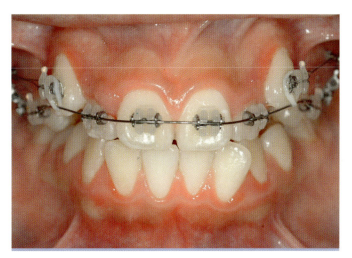

Fig. 2.37

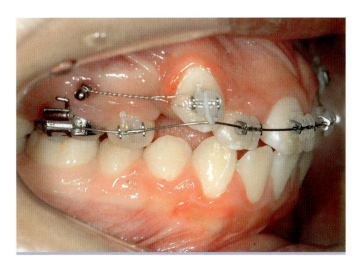

Fig. 2.38

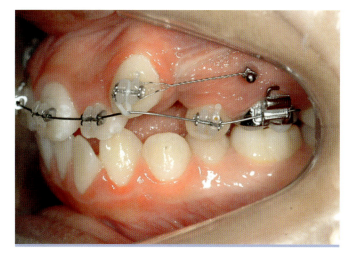

Fig. 2.39

Figs 2.37, 2.38 & 2.39 Canine retraction in the initial stage of treatment with absolute anchorage using miniscrews. The line of force is parallel to the orthodontic archwire, preventing the generation of vertical components.

the overbite, the line of force application should be changed by using a larger hook, welded to the mesial of the canines. This hook should be made with .019/.025 rectangular stainless steel archwire, and should be level with the miniscrew. The line of force application should be parallel to the orthodontic archwire (Figs 2.40, 2.41 & 2.42). When the line of force action is applied parallel to the orthodontic archwire, the direction of tooth movement will be parallel to the archwire (Fig. 2.43).

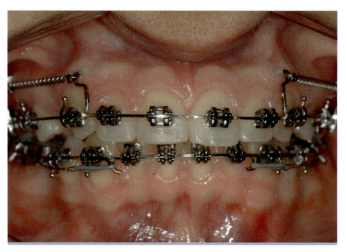

Fig. 2.40

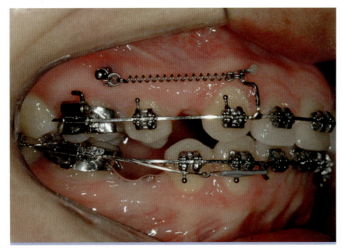

Fig. 2.41

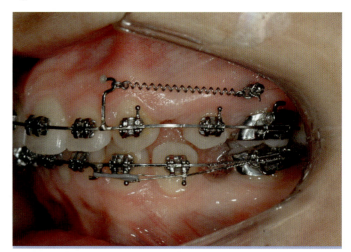

Fig. 2.42

Figs 2.40, 2.41 & 2.42 Space closure stage of treatment showing control of overbite. Hooks are prewelded to the mesial of the canines at the same height as the miniscrew. The line of force is parallel to the orthodontic archwire.

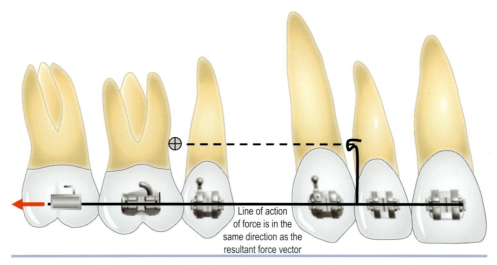

Line of action of force is in the same direction as the resultant force vector

Fig. 2.43 The line of force action is parallel to the archwire, creating a resultant in the same direction. This should be done in cases where the overbite is under control.

Class II treatment with molar distalization using miniscrews

Molar distalization using miniscrews

Class II malocclusions have always been a challenge in orthodontics, particularly in adult patients, as the Class II pattern prevails in these patients. These malocclusions are dento-skeletal in nature and can be due to maxillary protrusion or mandibular retrusion or a combination of mandibular retrusion and maxillary protrusion.

Class II malocclusions can be treated with headgear appliances, functional appliances, Class II elastics, and intraoral devices such as the Pendulum, Distal Jet, Nance button along with springs, etc. These appliances all demand cooperation from, and occasionally cause discomfort to, the patient. In addition to this, they are difficult to keep clean and biomechanical control is not easy.

One of the main difficulties in orthodontics has been the treatment of unilateral Class II malocclusions, especially in adult patients, as existing appliances do not allow unproblematic application of sectional biomechanics. However, now with miniscrews it is possible to integrate anchorage devices with the fixed orthodontic appliances. Thus, during molar distalization,[9] force application can be more predictable. Patient comfort and hygiene are also greatly improved due to the reduction in attachments used to apply the biomechanics. In Class II cases that require molar distalization, the site of insertion of the miniscrew should be occlusogingival, mesial to the first molars within the keratinized gingiva, concurring with the WALA ridge established by Andrews[10] (Figs 2.44 & 2.45). The interradicular space between the roots of the first molar and the second premolar, as well as the height of the alveolar bone crest, should be verified with periapical radiographs prior to the insertion. If there is insufficient space, it should be opened up by bonding the second premolar bracket in a counter-angulated position to move the roots mesially (see Fig. 2.24). The miniscrew recommended for distalizing molars in Class II cases is the 8 mm length screw. The force applied should be 250 g.

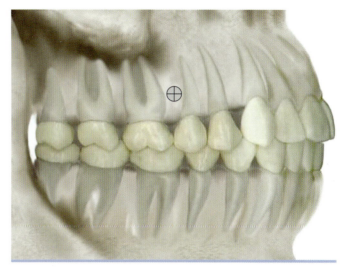

Fig. 2.44

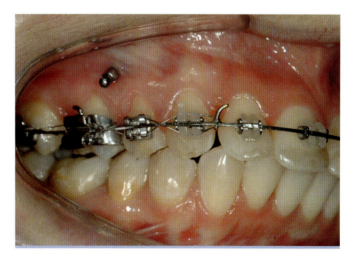

Fig. 2.45

Figs 2.44 & 2.45 Correct positioning of the miniscrew in Class II cases to distalize the molar – close to the center of resistance of the teeth or the WALA ridge.

There are two ways of distalizing the molars. The first is to use the fixed appliance without an auxiliary tube on the upper molars. In this case, a jig should be made with stiff .022 round stainless steel archwire, applying the force to the mesial of the molars (Figs 2.46, 2.47 & 2.48). The resulting force vectors do not allow full control over molar tipping, e.g. the molar may show more distal tipping. The angulation of the molar root is controlled by the main archwire. In this stage of treatment, the patient should have a .019/.025 rectangular archwire, which has been reduced posteriorly. The second option is to distalize the molars

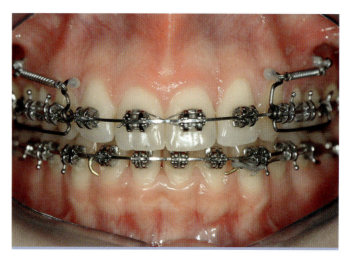

Fig. 2.46

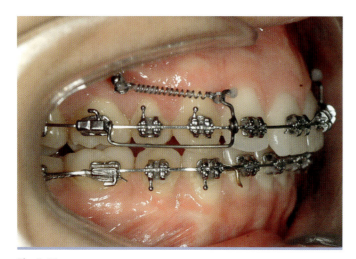

Fig. 2.47

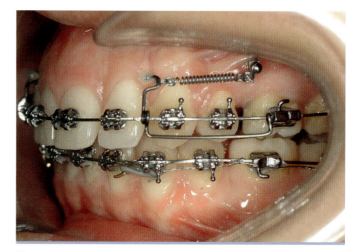

Fig. 2.48

Figs 2.46, 2.47 & 2.48 When single tubes are used on the molars, they can be distalized by using a jig made of .022 rectangular stainless steel wire.

using an auxiliary tube which has been positioned on the gingival aspect of the band or the bonded tube. Figures 2.49 & 2.50 show an adult patient in whom right upper molar distalization was planned with an auxiliary tube. A force of approximately 150 g should be applied immediately after the appliance is set up for 20 days and subsequently increased to 250 g.

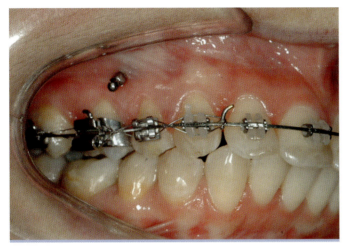

Fig. 2.49

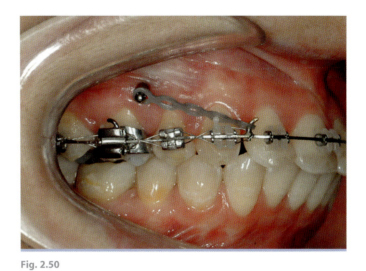

Fig. 2.50

Figs 2.49 & 2.50 Upper first molar band with gingival tube for distalization. Figure 2.18 shows the force of approximately 150 g being applied for the first 20 days.

The jig is built with .019/.025 rectangular stainless steel archwire, going from the mesial or distal of the canines to the auxiliary tube. At this point in the treatment, the clinician can commence molar distalization while monitoring the vertical changes. In patients with normal vertical dimensions, the jig should be placed at the same height as the miniscrew (Fig. 2.51). In normal overbite cases, the anterior segment of the jig should lie inferior to the miniscrew (Fig. 2.52). In deep bite cases, the jig should be placed below the height of the miniscrew, and, in anterior open bite cases, the anterior attachment point of the jig should be superior the miniscrew (Fig. 2.53). Placing the auxiliary tube closer to the center of resistance of the tooth and fitting the jig into the tube allows better molar tip control, and improved guided

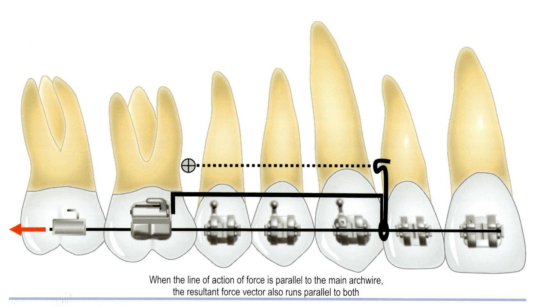

When the line of action of force is parallel to the main archwire, the resultant force vector also runs parallel to both

Fig. 2.51 When the line of force is at the same level as the resultant vector, the tooth movement will be in line with the archwire.

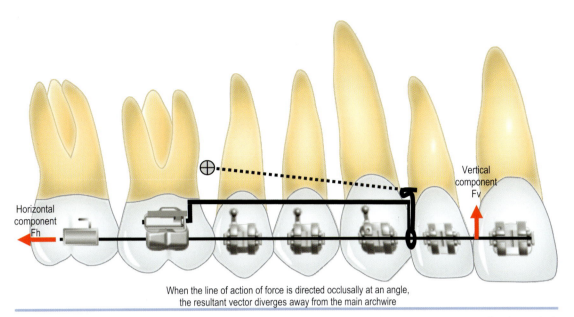

When the line of action of force is directed occlusally at an angle,
the resultant vector diverges away from the main archwire

Fig. 2.52 When the point of application of force is occlusal to the miniscrew, vertical components are created in the cervical direction.

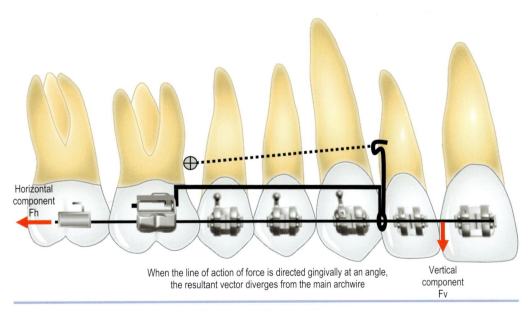

When the line of action of force is directed gingivally at an angle,
the resultant vector diverges from the main archwire

Fig. 2.53 When the point of application of force is cervical to the miniscrew, vertical components are created in the occlusal direction.

translation of the tooth. In this stage of treatment, if a conventional appliance is used, the premolars and the canines should be laced with metal ligatures to allow the natural distal movement of these teeth. In cases requiring unilateral distalization, the archwire should have a hook mesial to the canine on the opposite side (Figs 2.54, 2.55 & 2.56). The force applied to

distalize the upper molars should be approximately 250 g and continuous. There should be no hook on the side on which the distalization is being done to make fitting the jig easier. In cases of bilateral molar distalization, archwire hooks are best avoided to prevent interference with jig action (Figs 2.57, 2.58 & 2.59).

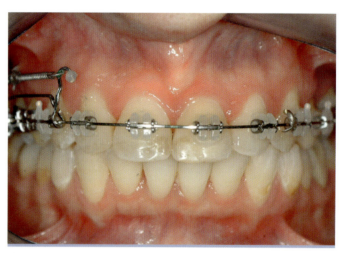

Fig. 2.54

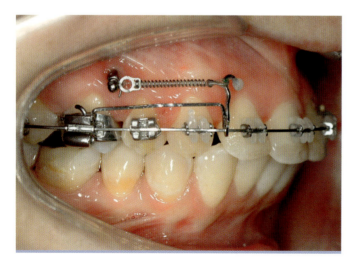

Fig. 2.55

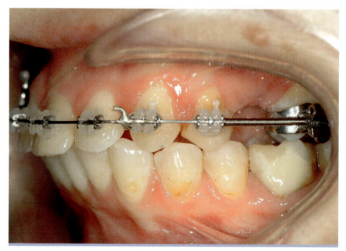

Fig. 2.56

Figs 2.54, 2.55 & 2.56 Unilateral right Class II case at the beginning of molar distalization using a jig fabricated of a .019/.025 rectangular stainless steel wire. On the left side, the archwire has been stabilized by tying a ligature from the brass hook on the archwire to the canine bracket.

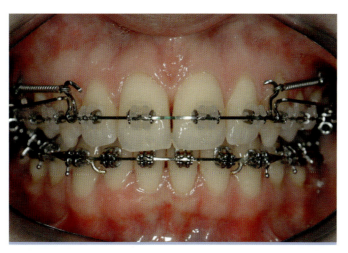

Fig. 2.57

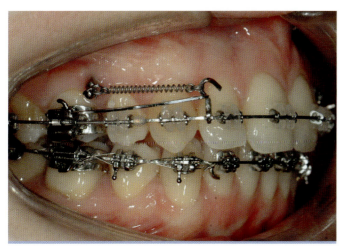

Fig. 2.58

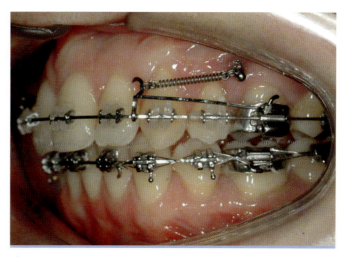

Fig. 2.59

Figs 2.57, 2.58 & 2.59 Bilateral Class II case with Clarity™ SL Self-Ligating Appliance. There are no prewelded hooks on the archwire for ease of molar distalization with jigs (.019/.025 rectangular stainless steel wire).

Anchorage considerations after molar distalization

The upper molar position should be overcorrected by about 1–2 mm distally, as seen in Figure 2.60, to allow for anchorage loss during the retraction of the premolars and anterior teeth. To enable planning of the type of anchorage to be used, the distal tipping of molars should be monitored during the distal movement. Ideally, there should be good tip control of the molars to allow sliding mechanics. At this stage of treatment, the archwire should slide freely through the slots of buccal tubes of first and second molars.

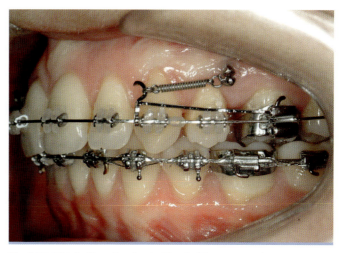

Fig. 2.60 Distalization of molars to Class I with overcorrection.

A new miniscrew should be inserted close to the molar root 3 months after the end of molar distalization. During this period of time, no active treatment should be undertaken to allow the formation of alveolar bone mesial to the molars. If this option is chosen, the clinician should fabricate an intermediate .018 round stainless steel archwire, with omega loops to the mesial of the molars, to prevent the molars from moving mesially (Figs 2.61, 2.62 & 2.63). An alternative option is to use a palatal bar to preserve

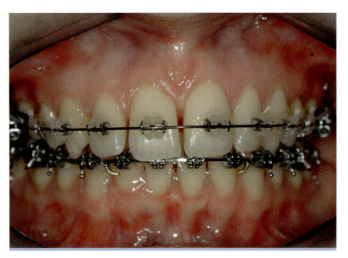

Fig. 2.61

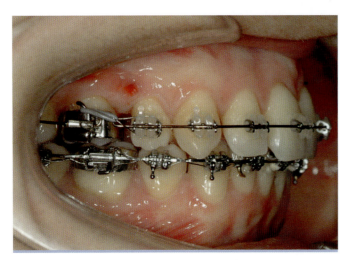

Fig. 2.62

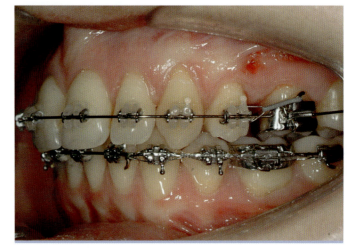

Fig. 2.63

Figs 2.61, 2.62 & 2.63 A .018 round stainless steel archwire with omega loops. This archwire should be kept in place for 3 months.

the anchorage. With this option, the clinician should pay close attention to unwanted anchorage loss. The last option is to use headgear for 4 hours a day, applying Class II mechanics with intermaxillary elastics. This option will, of course, depend on patient cooperation (Figs 2.64, 2.65, 2.66 & 2.67).

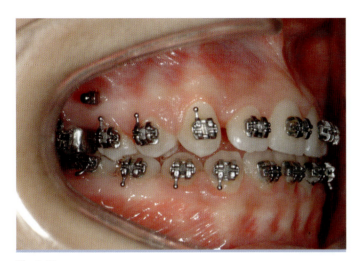

Fig. 2.64

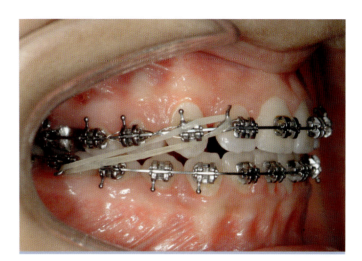

Fig. 2.65

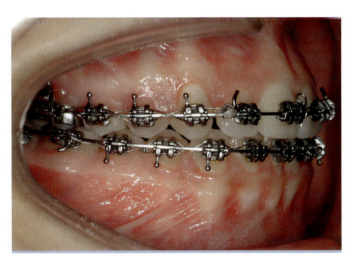

Fig. 2.66

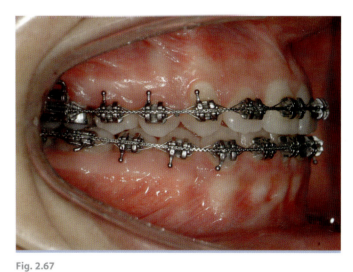

Fig. 2.67

Figs 2.64, 2.65, 2.66 & 2.67 Stage of treatment after the distalization of the molar using miniscrews, using a 019/.025 rectangular stainless steel archwire and Class II elastics; end of the retraction stage with passive lacebacks; detailing stage with .019/.025 braided archwire.

Space closure mechanics

Once the anchorage system involving the molars is established, the mechanics for closing the premolar spaces and retracting the anterior segment should be started.[11] In this stage of treatment, the patient should have a .019/.025 rectangular stainless steel archwire engaged, with prewelded hooks mesial to the canines and at the same height as the miniscrews. With this appliance set-up, the line of action of the force applied will be parallel to the archwire, which avoids creation of vertical moments, and minimizes the friction generated between the archwire and the bracket slot. The retraction system applied to close the spaces can consist of Nitinol springs or elastic modules attached to metal ligatures (Figs 2.68, 2.69 & 2.70). The space

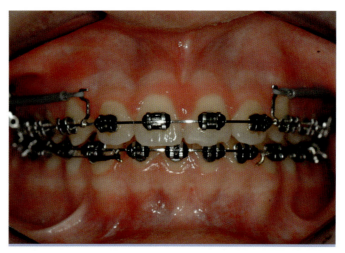

Fig. 2.68

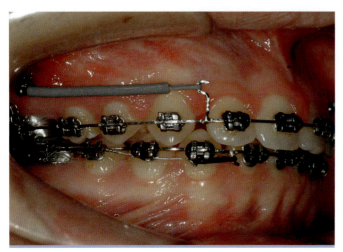

Fig. 2.69

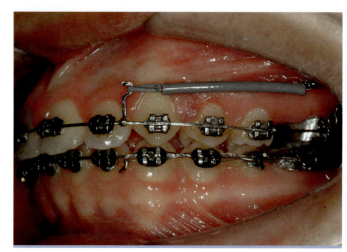

Fig. 2.70

Figs 2.68, 2.69 & 2.70 Distalization of the premolars and retraction of the anterior segment with miniscrews reinserted closer to the roots of the first molars.

closure system using elastic modules and metal ligatures, with 3 mm activation, provides an initial force of 370 g in the first 24 hours, which reduces to an average force of 193 g over the following 28 days (Fig. 2.71).

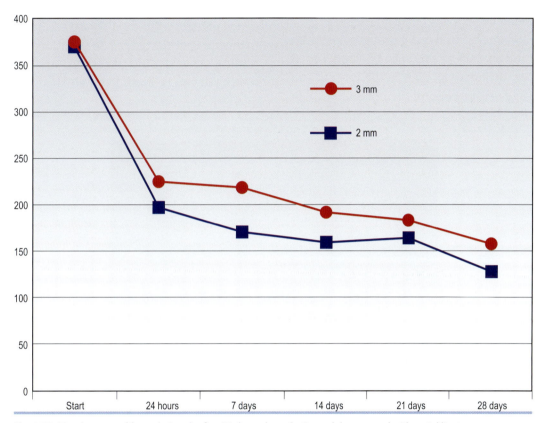

Fig. 2.71 The decrease of force during the first 28 days when elastic modules are used with metal ligatures.

After completion of space closure, the retraction system should be kept in place for 1 month to allow the roots to express the angulation built into the brackets, preventing relapse. After this stage of treatment, figure-of-eight metal ligatures (passive lacebacks) should be inserted from the hook on the mesial of the canine to the last posterior tooth on each side, which transfers the torque in the appliance to the roots of the teeth. This stage of treatment is called torque settling (see Fig. 2.66).

Details and finishing

The last stage of treatment is finishing and detailing, at which point many aspects of the orthodontic treatment should be reviewed and observed. This includes evaluating and verifying: the position of the molars, premolars and canines and the interarch relationship at each level; the arch form; root paralleling, cephalometric and facial profile goals; the contact points; the absence or presence of rotations; the curve of Spee; the curve of Wilson; the vertical and horizontal overbite of the canines; the functional goals in relation to the occlusion; and temporomandibular joint function. After such an evaluation, the process of settling the occlusion may be started with .019/.025 rectangular braided archwires and 3/16 (4 oz) triangular elastics worn fulltime, 24 hours a day, for 15 days and only at night for a further 20 days. Prior to the placement of the braided archwires, place a figure-of-eight .008 steel ligature from molar to molar to ensure that the spaces do not reopen during settling. After settling the occlusion, the orthodontic treatment can be considered finished (Figs 2.72, 2.73 & 2.74).

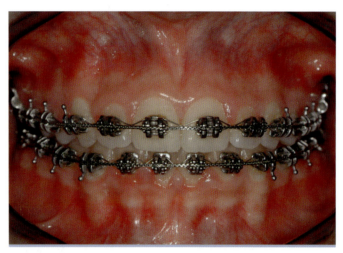

Fig. 2.72

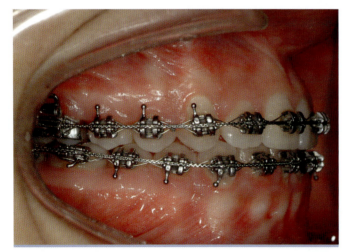

Fig. 2.73

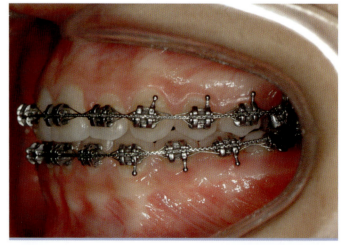

Fig. 2.74

Figs 2.72, 2.73 & 2.74 Final stage of settling the occlusion with a .019/.025 braided archwire. Before engaging the archwire, a .008 figure-of-eight ligature was placed.

Intrusion of teeth using miniscrews

Miniscrews are highly efficient in the intrusion of teeth in the posterior and anterior segments. When the goal is to intrude teeth, the site of insertion of the miniscrew should be carefully established. This is frequently above the center of resistance in the case of the maxilla, and below the center of resistance in the case of the mandible. These areas are closer to the tooth apices with greater interradicular space, making insertion of miniscrews less risky in terms of damage to the roots.

Intrusion of the molars

The use of miniscrews for the intrusion of teeth in the posterior segment is indicated in many situations, such as: intrusion of over-erupted molars[12] and premolars due to the early loss of teeth in the opposing arch prior to prosthetic rehabilitation; intrusion of molars in patients with posterior vertical excess to correct anterior open bites;[13] and in cases with buccal crossbite with upper and lower molar extrusion.

In cases requiring molar and premolar intrusion, torque is controlled with a palatal bar or with the addition of compensating torque to the archwire. For better control of intrusion of molars, two miniscrews should be used. One of these miniscrews should be inserted buccally in the mandible, and the other near the palatal surface of the corresponding maxillary tooth.

Buccal molar crossbite with associated extrusion of teeth is difficult to treat with conventional orthodontics, as there is no occlusion with the teeth in the opposing arch (Figs 2.75, 2.76 & 2.77). Although there is a 1 mm overbite in the buccal crossbite region, there will be a 3 mm opening on the incisor area. The use of cross-elastics is not indicated in this situation, as they often cause over-extrusion of teeth. The use of miniscrews sited palatal to the upper molars and buccal to the lower teeth is highly recommended as it enables the intrusion of teeth and at the same time enables control of torque, palatal tipping of the upper molars and buccal tipping of the lower molars.

The first step in this treatment is intrusion of the molars (Figs 2.78 & 2.79) and the second stage is alignment and leveling with the use of horizontal springs and addition of torque to the archwire (Figs 2.80, 2.81 & 2.82).

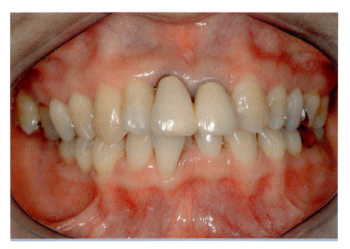

Fig. 2.75

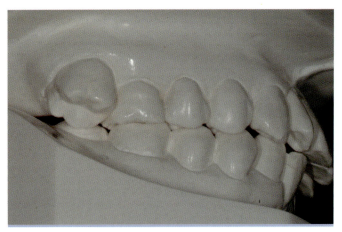

Fig. 2.76

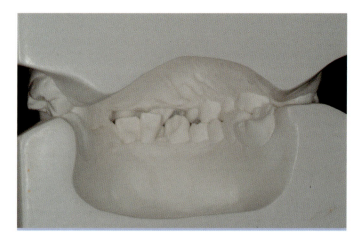

Fig. 2.77

Figs 2.75, 2.76 & 2.77 Malocclusion with molar crossbite and extrusion.

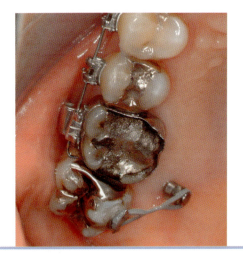

Fig. 2.78

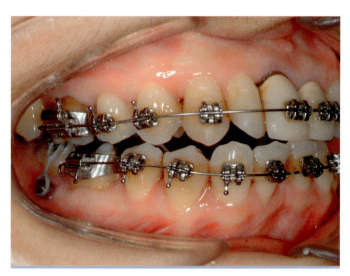

Fig. 2.79

Figs 2.78 & 2.79 The miniscrew was inserted buccally in the mandible, and palatally in the maxilla, to allow intrusion of the molars.

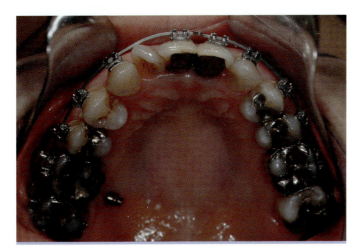

Fig. 2.80

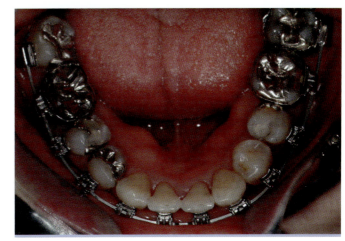

Fig. 2.81

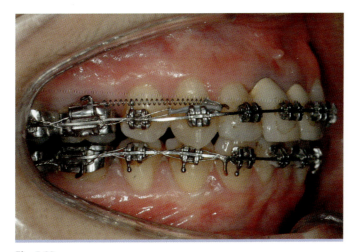

Fig. 2.82

Figs 2.80, 2.81 & 2.82 In the maxilla, the molar was intruded. In the mandible, miniscrews were used in the treatment.

Intrusion of lower incisors

Major discrepancies in overbite or vertical height can compromise orthodontic treatment results and should be treated prior to resolution of horizontal discrepancies. Anterior tooth intrusion by conventional orthodontic procedures is carried out with the use of a reverse curve orthodontic archwire or the Ricketts utility arch.[14] However, using these auxiliaries extends the treatment time, generates unwanted moments and causes the molars to tip buccally and distally. Proclination of the incisor teeth is a common occurrence when correcting the overbite. This happens due to the nature of the reverse curve archwire, which creates friction during the sliding mechanics.

The intrusion of the anterior teeth with sectional forces with miniscrews does not compromise the other arch segments during the orthodontic treatment. This approach is beneficial for orthodontic biomechanics, in particular in adult patients (Figs 2.83 & 2.84).

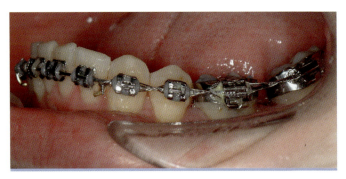

Fig. 2.83

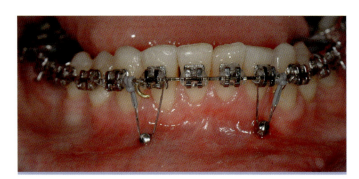

Fig. 2.84

Figs 2.83 & 2.84 Figure 2.83 shows an arch with a severe curve of Spee, which is difficult to correct using a reverse curve .019/.025 rectangular archwire. Figure 2.84 shows miniscrews inserted to the distal of the lateral incisors and an intrusive force applied with .009 ligatures and elastic modules.

The incisors should be intruded when the treatment is in the rectangular archwire stage to maintain torque control. Depending on the initial inclination of the incisors, labial root torque should be added to control the labial inclination of the crowns (Figs 2.85 & 2.86). This stage in the treatment

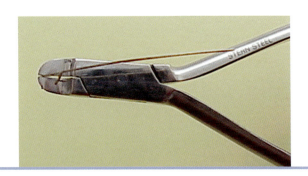

Fig. 2.85

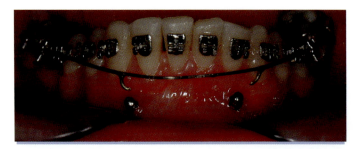

Fig. 2.86

Figs 2.85 & 2.86 Figure 2.85 shows the orthodontic archwire with labial root torque in the lower incisor region to control the labial inclination of the incisor crowns. Figure 2.86 shows the archwire with labial root torque in situ.

(Figs 2.87, 2.88 & 2.89) should be carefully monitored to achieve an ideal vertical overbite.

The reverse curve archwire should be removed after a few weeks following the correction of the overbite (Figs 2.90, 2.91 & 2.92) and not immediately. The

miniscrews can be removed at the end of treatment, in the finishing and detailing stages (Figs 2.93, 2.94 & 2.95). The full appliance should only be removed after verifying the stability of the orthodontic result (Figs 2.96, 2.97 & 2.98).

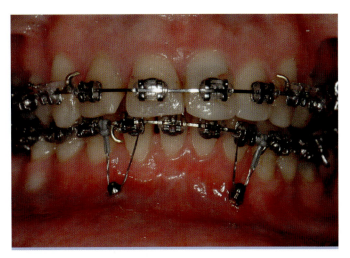

Fig. 2.87

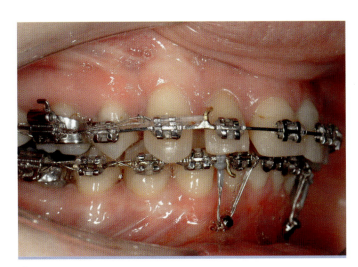

Fig. 2.88

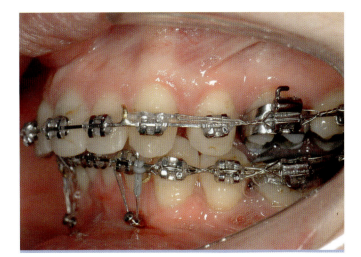

Fig. 2.89

Figs 2.87, 2.88 & 2.89 A .019/.025 rectangular archwire with torque control of the lower incisors. Miniscrews with force applied using metal ligatures in combination with elastic modules.

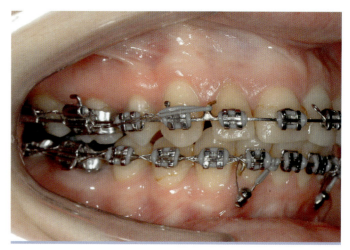

Figs 2.90, 2.91 & 2.92 Satisfactory correction of the overbite without any undesired tooth movement in the remaining segments.

Fig. 2.90

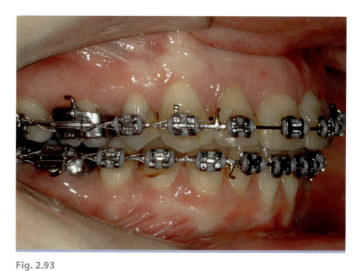

Figs 2.93, 2.94 & 2.95 Final stage of treatment without the miniscrews. The spaces have been closed in the upper arch.

Fig. 2.93

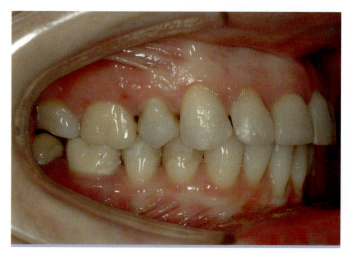

Figs 2.96, 2.97 & 2.98 Treatment finished with appliance removal. The centerlines and the overbite have been corrected, with a Class II molar relationship on the right side and Class I molar relationship on the left side.

Fig. 2.96

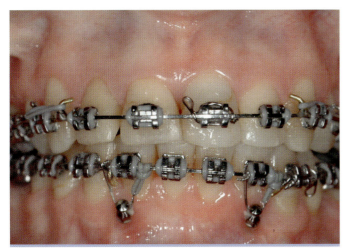

Fig. 2.91

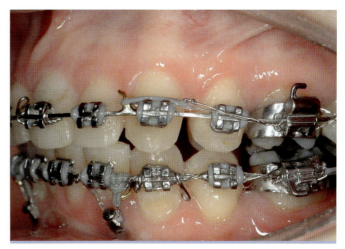

Fig. 2.92

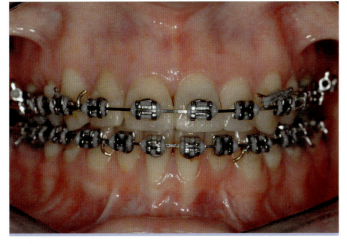

Fig. 2.94

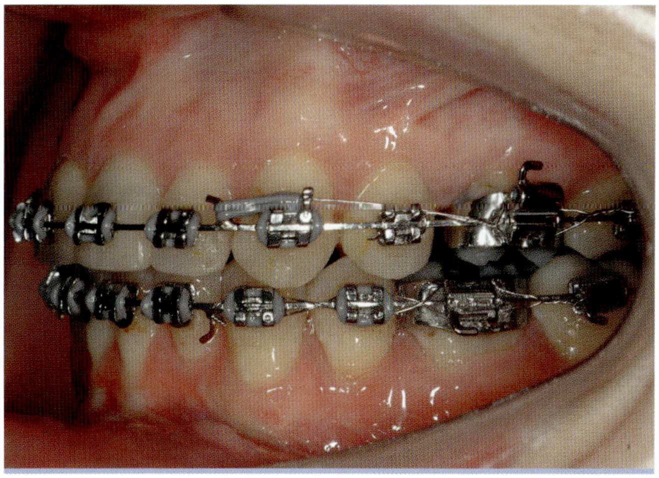

Fig. 2.95

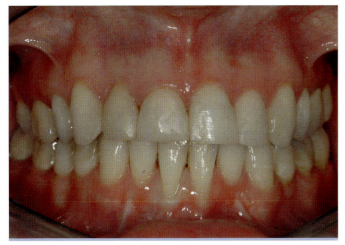

Fig. 2.97

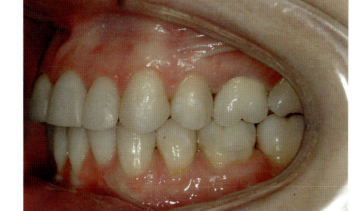

Fig. 2.98

Intrusion of upper incisors

One of the characteristics of brachyfacial patients is a deep overbite, which is the result of extrusion of the upper or lower incisors. In patients with upper incisor extrusion, with no possibility of appliance placement in the lower arch, conventional treatment is initiated with a stainless steel archwire with a bend to the mesial of the molar, with a reverse curve archwire or with a Ricketts utility arch.[14] Usually, these mechanics create a force moment at the molars, which tips these teeth distally, making sliding mechanics difficult (Fig. 2.99). Miniscrews are an excellent option in these cases – the light forces generated by the mechanics are complemented with a guided continuous force established at the miniscrew (Fig. 2.100). The miniscrew should be inserted between the two central incisors, above the center of resistance of the teeth and

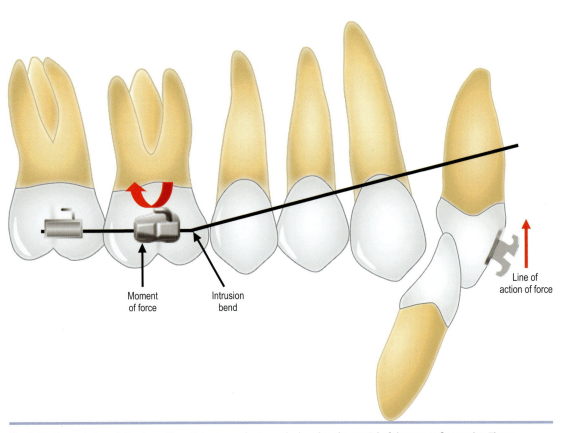

Moment of force

Intrusion bend

Line of action of force

Fig. 2.99 Upper incisors intrusion with an intrusive archwire and a bend to the mesial of the upper first molar. These mechanics tip the molar distally.

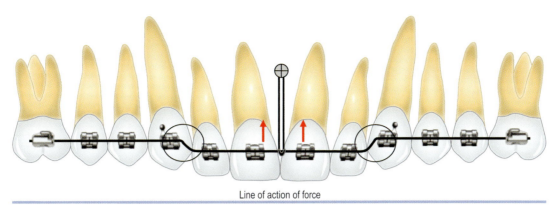

Line of action of force

Fig. 2.100 A very low force generated by the biomechanics and a continuous force produced by the miniscrew.

close to the teeth apices (Fig. 2.101).[15] Another option is to insert two miniscrews to the distal of the lateral incisors.[16] In this approach, it is advisable to apply the intrusive mechanics with a rectangular archwire in place to control the inclination of the incisors.

When intruding the teeth, the angulation of teeth can be affected by the moments established by this kind of mechanics. Thus, the anterior teeth, canine to canine, should be laced back with a .008 ligature (Fig. 2.102).

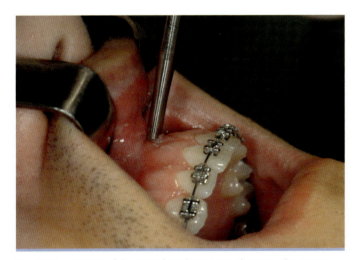

Fig. 2.101 Insertion of the 6 mm length miniscrew between the upper central incisors, just above the center of resistance.

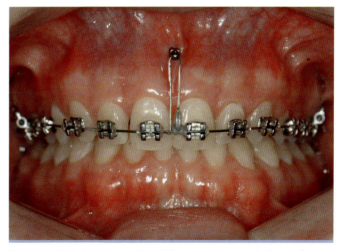

Fig. 2.102 Initiating the intrusion of the upper incisor with the low force delivered via the archwire and a continuous force generated by the miniscrew.

Mesialization and uprighting of molars using miniscrews

Mesialization of molars, without changing the position of the anterior teeth, may be required in a number of orthodontic cases. This procedure is almost impossible without the use of miniscrews, as the alternative is to use the anterior teeth as an anchorage system to protract the molars, which is difficult to achieve. Another method of mesializing the molars is by using reverse pull headgear – one which demands exemplary cooperation and severely compromises facial esthetics during treatment.

There are many other situations in which miniscrews can be recommended. For instance, in patients with agenesis of second premolars with a good cephalometric position of the incisor teeth (Figs 2.103, 2.104, 2.105 & 2.106), miniscrews can be used as an anchorage system to mesialize the upper and the lower

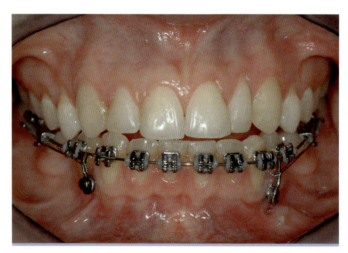

Fig. 2.103

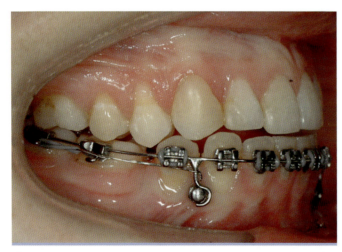

Fig. 2.104

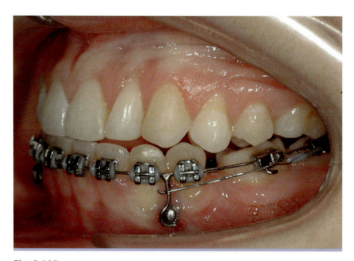

Fig. 2.105

Figs 2.103, 2.104 & 2.105 Insertion of the miniscrew to the mesial of the lower first premolars and a long hook welded to the archwire, which is being supported by the miniscrew. Force application is indirect and parallel to the archwire.

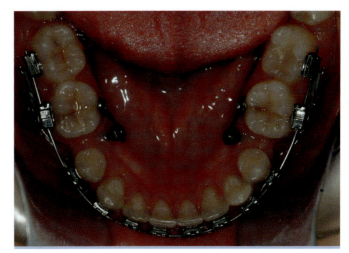

Fig. 2.106

Figs 2.106 Occlusal view with miniscrews inserted to the distal of the first premolars for applying lingual retraction in association with buccal mechanics.

molars[17] to close the spaces created by the absent teeth without affecting the inclination of the incisors. In such cases, molar mesialization should be initiated after all the present premolars have erupted. Miniscrews are inserted to the mesial of the first premolar to allow the biomechanical force direction to be parallel to the main archwire, thus preventing undesired vertical movement. The treatment is finished in a Class II molar relationship in cases with upper premolar agenesis, and in a Class III molar relationship in cases with lower premolar agenesis (Figs 2.107, 2.108 & 2.109).

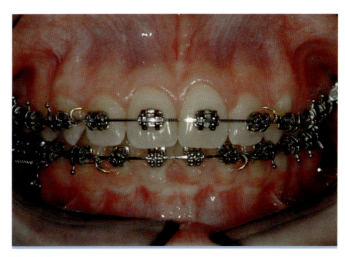

Fig. 2.107

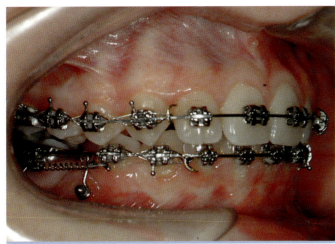

Fig. 2.108

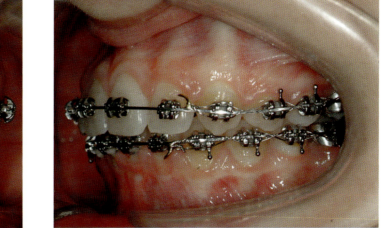

Fig. 2.109

Figs 2.107, 2.108 & 2.109 **Agenesis of the lower right second premolar. A miniscrew was inserted distal to the first premolar and a force** arm was built with a 0.6 mm round stainless steel archwire which was welded to the rectangular archwire. The force was applied to the mesial of molar, parallel to the main archwire.

One of the chief benefits of the use of miniscrews in contemporary orthodontics is seen in adult patients with early loss of posterior teeth, in particular when there are no first molars.[18] With the loss of the posterior teeth, several uncontrolled tooth movements occur, such as distalization and rotation of premolars, mesialization and rotation or tipping of molars and extrusion of antagonist teeth. In such cases, the treatment goals require initial uprighting of posterior teeth, followed by either prosthetic rehabilitation or space closure by mesialization. Molar uprighting always necessitates carrying out difficult maneuvers with uprighting springs, additional archwires, cantilevers, etc. Every orthodontic technique for uprighting molars creates vertical force components that encourage extrusion of the molars, resulting in partial or complete open bites. The use of miniscrews to upright the molars[19] enables sectional control of treatment as only desirable force moments are introduced into the biomechanics, thereby maintaining control over unwanted molar extrusion (Fig. 2.110).

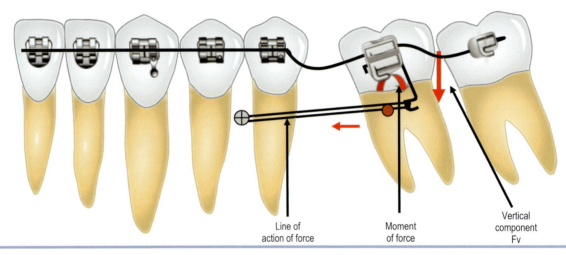

Line of action of force

Moment of force

Vertical component Fv

Fig. 2.110 Molar uprighting with a molar band with tube attachment and a force arm that is arising distal to the tube and a miniscrew inserted to the mesial of the first premolar. The line of action of the resultant force is parallel to the main archwire.

References

1. Brito V S Jr, Ursi, W J S 2006 O aparelho pré-ajustado: sua evolução e suas prescrições. Revista Dental Press de Ortodontia e Ortopedia Facial 11:104–156

2. Lee J S, Kim J K, Park Y C, Vanarsdall R L 2007 Applications of orthodontic mini-implants. Quintessence, Chicago

3. Trevisi H 2007 SmartClip™: tratamento ortodôntico com sistema de aparelho autoligado – conceito e biomecânica. Elsevier, Rio de Janeiro

4. Kim J H, Ahn S J, Chang Y I 2005 Histomorphometric and mechanical analyses of the drill-free screw as orthodontic anchorage. American Journal of Orthodontics and Dentofacial Orthopedics 128:190–194

5. Villela H, Bezerra F, Labossiére M J 2006 Micro parafuso ortodôntico de titânio auto perfurante (MPO): Novo protocolo cirúrgico e atuais perspectivas clínicas. Innovations Implant Journal 1:46–53

6. Marassi C, Leal A, Herdy J L, Chianelli O, Sobriera D 2005 O uso de mini-implantes como método auxiliar do tratamento ortodôntico. Ortodontia SPO 38:256–265

7. Zanelato A C T, Trevisi H, Zanelato R C T, Zanelato A C T, Trevisi R C 2006 Análise da Movimentação Dentária (VTO dentário). Revista Clínica de Ortodontia 5:59–65

8. Morea C, Dominguez G C, Wuo Ado V, Tortamano A 2005 Surgical guide for optimal positioning of miniimplants. Journal of Clinical Orthodontics 39:317–321

9. Seling-Min L, Ryoon-Ki H 2008 Distal movement of maxillary molars using a lever-arm and mini-implant system. Angle Orthodontist 78:167–175

10. Andrews L F, Andrews W A 1995 Syllabus of Andrews philosophy and techniques, 5th ed. Lawrence F Andrews Foundation, San Diego

11. Marassi C, Marassi C 2008 Mini-implantes ortodônticos como auxiliares da fase de retração anterior. Revista Dental Press de Ortodontia e Ortopedia Facial 13:57–75

12. Villela H M, Bezerra F J B, Lemos L N, Pessoa S M L 2008 Maxillary molar intrusion using self-drilling titanium orthodontic micro screws. Revista Clinica de Ortodontia 7:52–64

13. Chunlei X, Xian G Z, Xing W 2007 Micro screw anchorage in skeletal anterior open-bite treatment. Angle Orthodontist 77:47–56

14. Ricketts R M 2003 Conceitos de mecânica e biomecânica. Artes Gráficas, Goiânia

15. Costa A, Raffaini M, Melsen B 1998 Miniscrews as orthodontic anchorage: a preliminary report. International Journal of Adult Orthodontics and Orthognathic Surgery 13:201–209

16. Carano A, Velo S, Leone P, Siciliani G 2005 Clinical applications of the miniscrew anchorage system. Journal of Clinical Orthodontics 39:9–42

17. Janson M, Silva D A F 2008 Mesialização de molares com ancoragem em mini-implantes. Revista Dental Press de Ortodontia e Ortopedia Facial 13:88–94

18. Kyung S H, Choi J H, Park Y C 2003 Miniscrew anchorage used to protract lower second molars into first molar extraction sites. Journal of Clinical Orthodontics 37:575–579

19. Bicalho R F, Bicalho J S, Laboissière J M 2009 Indirect skeletal anchorage used to upright mandibular molars. Revista Clinica de Ortodontia Dental Press 8:63–68

Chapter 2 Clinical case

Name: AC
Sex: Female
Age: 19 years
Facial pattern: Brachyfacial
Skeletal pattern: Class II
Treatment time: 30 months

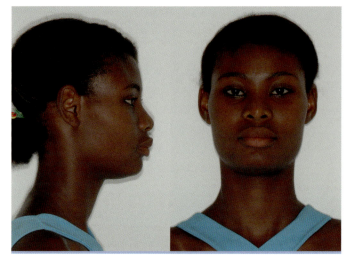

Fig. 2.111   Fig. 2.112

Diagnosis

Brachyfacial skeletal pattern and Class II dental malocclusion. Deep overbite and crossbite of the first premolars. Severe proclination of the upper and the lower incisors and accentuated curve of Spee.

Treatment plan

The orthodontic treatment was carried out with upper first premolar extractions and miniscrew anchorage. The treatment was planned to be completed with a Class II molar relationship, with correction of the curve of Spee while controlling the proclination of the upper and the lower incisors.

Appliances

- Upper and lower SmartClip™ Self-Ligating Appliance
- Lingual arch
- Miniscrew to the mesial of the upper first molars

Figs 2.111 & 2.112
Pretreatment extraoral photographs showing the facial symmetry, the facial profile and a severe brachyfacial Class II malocclusion.

- Hawley retainer in the upper arch
- Fixed 3 × 3 retainer in the lower arch.

Case report

Brachyfacial patient with skeletal pattern and Class II malocclusion, presenting with a deep overbite, buccal crossbite of the upper first molars, marked proclination of the upper and lower incisors, increased overjet and accentuated curve of Spee.

The treatment plan was to extract the upper and lower third molars and place the SmartClip™ Self-Ligating Appliance in the upper arch. After initial alignment, the interradicular space between the upper second premolars and the first molars was opened with Nitinol springs to allow insertion of miniscrews.

In the lower arch, a lingual arch was bonded to maintain the existing spaces. Then, the SmartClip™ Self-Ligating Appliance was placed in the lower arch with a .014 round Nitinol superelastic archwire to initiate alignment as for the upper arch. This was completed with a .016 round Nitinol superelastic archwire and leveling was carried out with a .017/.025 rectangular Nitinol superelastic archwire and finished with a .019/.025 rectangular Nitinol archwire.

Miniscrews were inserted above the centers of resistance of the teeth to provide anchorage for correcting the deep overbite. The upper first premolars were extracted when the patient was in .019/.025 rectangular stainless steel archwires. Retraction of the upper anterior segment was initiated using sliding mechanics with Nitinol springs and hooks prewelded to the mesial of the canines.

For the correction of the curve of Spee, a reverse curve was applied to the lower .019/.025 rectangular archwire, with labial root torque to prevent lower incisor proclination. After the correction of the deep overbite, there was spatial advancement of the mandible, establishing the Class II overcorrection. The miniscrews were removed and the sliding mechanics continued with no additional anchorage requirements.

In the final stage of space closure, the versatility of the MBT™ philosophy was utilized. The upper and lower second molar tubes were changed, that is, the upper molars were fitted with lower second molar tubes of the opposite side. Re-leveling was done with a .018 round Nitinol archwire and finally a .019/.025 rectangular stainless steel archwire was inserted while closing the remaining spaces.

Finishing and details was carried out with .019/.025 rectangular braided archwires and 3/16 (4 oz) vertical elastics used at night time.

Retention involved use of a Hawley retainer in the upper arch and a 3 × 3 fixed retainer in the lower arch.

The treatment achieved functional movements with stability and improvement of the facial esthetics.

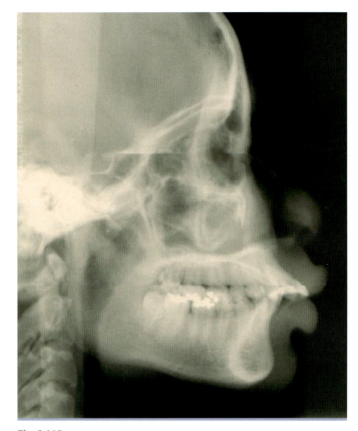

Figs 2.113, 2.114 & 2.115
Cephalometric radiograph, tracing and analysis, showing decreased vertical measurements and severe proclination of the upper and lower incisors.

Fig. 2.113

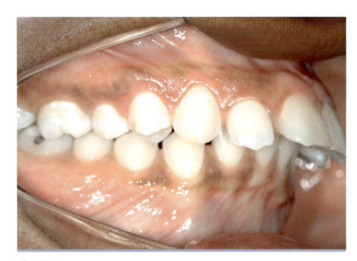

Figs 2.116, 2.117 & 2.118
Pretreatment intraoral photographs showing the Class II molar relationship, deep overbite and severe bimaxillary protrusion.

Fig. 2.116

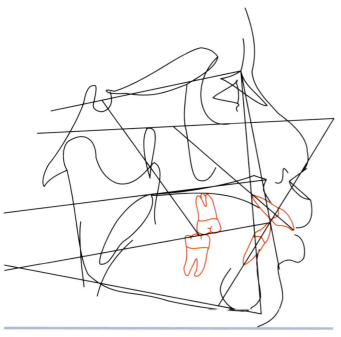

Fig. 2.114

SNA ∠	89º
SNB ∠	83º
ANB ∠	6º
A-N ⊥ FH	8 mm
Po-N ⊥ FH	4 mm
Wits	10 mm
GoGn SN ∠	20º
FH Md ∠	13º
Mx Md ∠	17º
U1 to A-Po	15 mm
L1 to A-Po	3 mm
U1 to Mx plane ∠	133º
L1 to Md plane ∠	112º
Facial analysis	
Nasolabial ∠	74º
NA ⊥ nose ∠	24 mm
Lip thickness	11.5 mm

Fig. 2.115

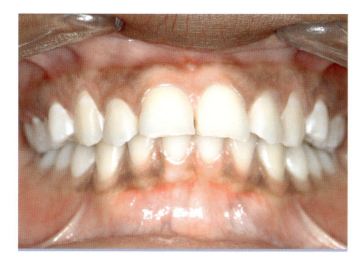

Fig. 2.117

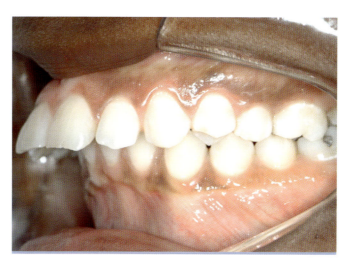

Fig. 2.118

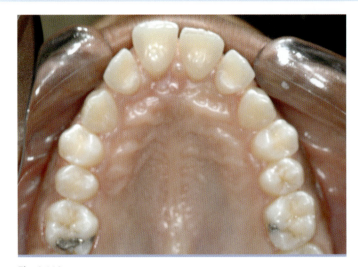

Fig. 2.119

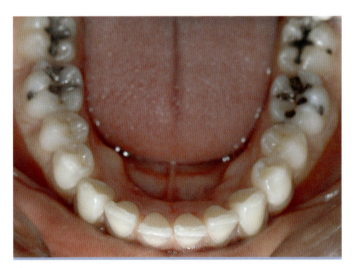

Fig. 2.120

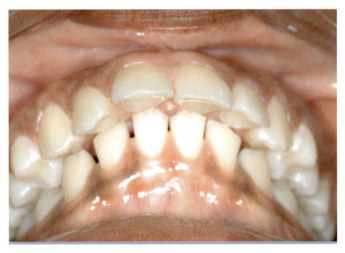

Figs 2.119, 2.120 & 2.121
Pretreatment occlusal views showing the upper and lower dental arches. Figure 2.121 shows the upper first premolars in buccal crossbite and the lower incisors in close contact with the palatal gingiva.

Fig. 2.121

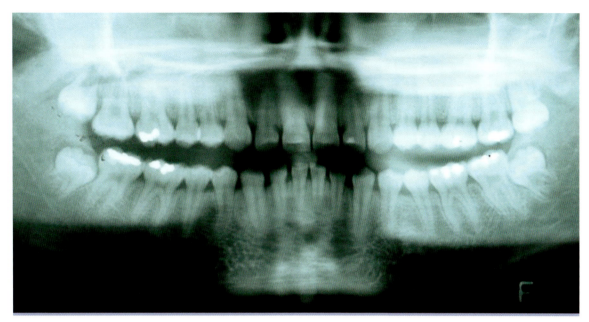

Fig. 2.122

Fig. 2.122
Panoramic radiograph showing the permanent dentition including the impacted lower third molars.

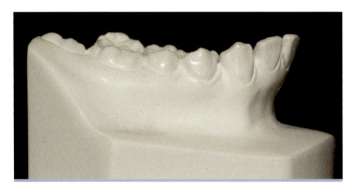

Fig. 2.123

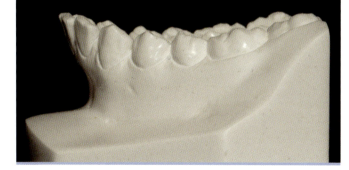

Fig. 2.124

Figs 2.123 & 2.124
Right and left lateral views of the pretreatment study models showing the accentuated curve of Spee.

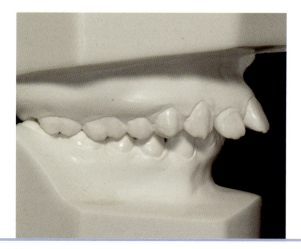

Figs 2.125, 2.126 & 2.127
Study models showing the molars in a Class II relationship and deep overbite with severe proclination of the upper and lower incisors.

Fig. 2.125

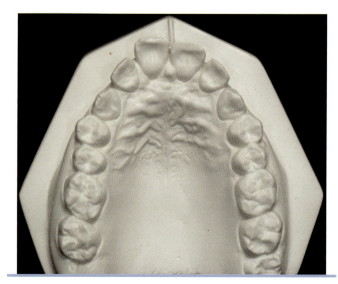

Fig. 2.128

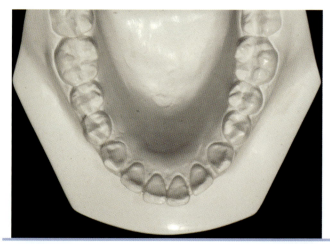

Figs 2.128 & 2.129
Occlusal view of the study models showing the spacing in the upper and lower aches and the straight teeth.

Fig. 2.129

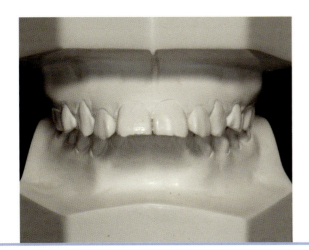

Fig. 2.126

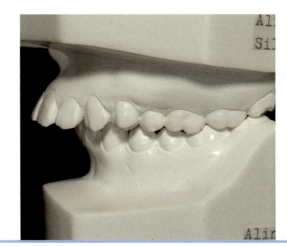

Fig. 2.127

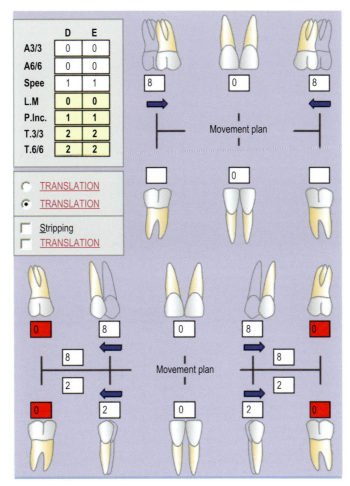

Fig. 2.130

Fig. 2.130

Orthodontic treatment planning using the dental VTO. The malocclusion requires absolute anchorage in the upper and lower arches with upper premolar extraction.

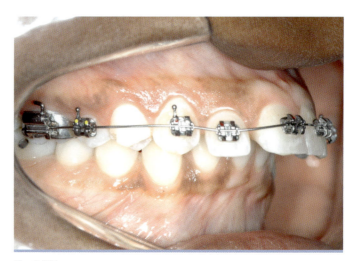

Fig. 2.131

Figs 2.131, 2.132 & 2.133
Appliance set-up in the upper arch with a .014 round Nitinol superelastic archwire, initiating the aligning stage of treatment. No brackets were placed on the first premolars.

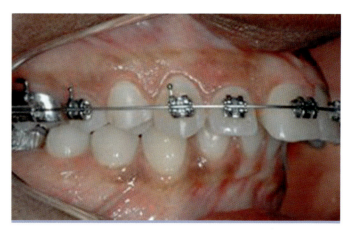

Fig. 2.134

Figs 2.134, 2.135 & 2.136
Finishing off the aligning and the leveling of the upper arch with a .017/.025 rectangular Nitinol archwire.

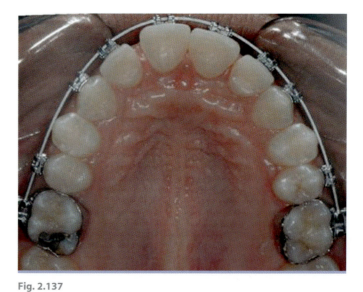

Fig. 2.137

Figs 2.137 & 2.138
Occlusal view of a .017/.025 rectangular Nitinol archwire in the upper arch, and a lingual arch in the lower arch, aiming to preserve the molar anchorage.

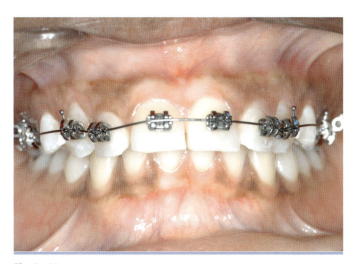

Fig. 2.132

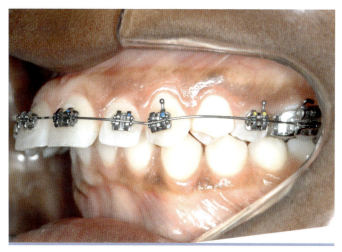

Fig. 2.133

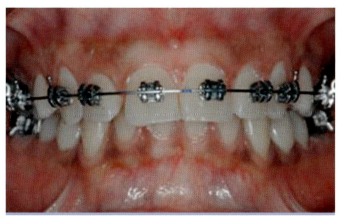

Fig. 2.135

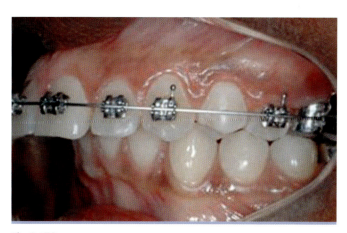

Fig. 2.136

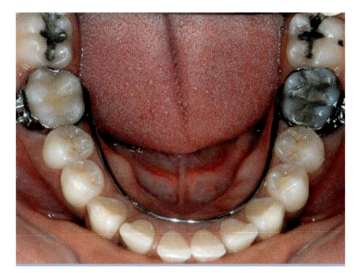

Fig. 2.138

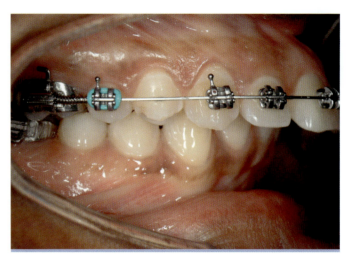

Fig. 2.139

Figs 2.139 & 2.140

Space creation for the miniscrews with open coil springs placed between the molar and the second premolar. An elastic module was placed on the premolar brackets to prevent rotation.

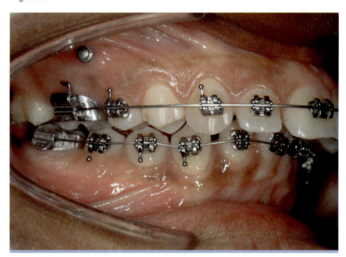

Fig. 2.141

Figs 2.141, 2.142 & 2.143

Miniscrew inserted to the mesial of the upper first molars, above the center of resistance of the teeth. SmartClip™ Self-Ligating Appliance on the lower arch with a .014 round Nitinol superelastic archwire starting the alignment stage.

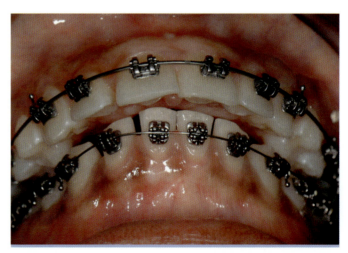

Fig. 2.144

Fig. 2.144

Overjet and overbite at the beginning of the leveling phase. The lower incisors are no longer touching the palatal gingiva.

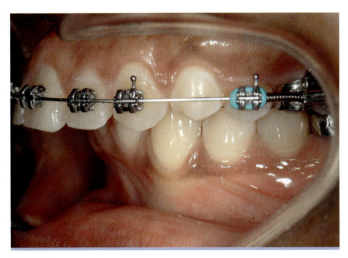

Fig. 2.140

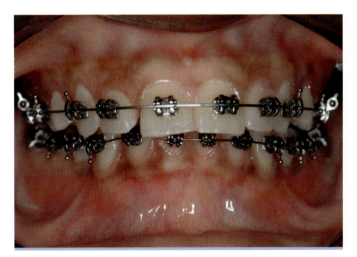

Fig. 2.142

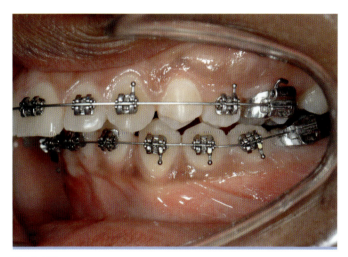

Fig. 2.143

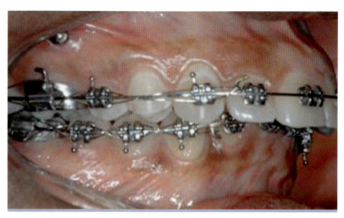

Figs 2.145, 2.146 & 2.147
Frontal and lateral views showing the end of leveling with .019/.025 rectangular stainless steel archwire. In this stage, passive lacebacks should be placed from the hooks welded to the mesial of the canines to the second molars, using .009 ligature wires.

Fig. 2.145

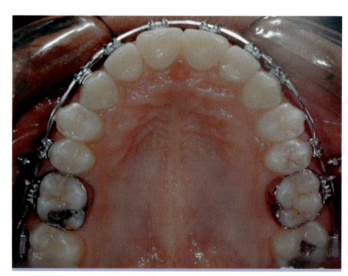

Figs 2.148 & 2.149
Occlusal view of the upper and lower arches, showing the alignment, leveling and the well-established dental arches. The lower lingual arch has been removed and lower anterior labial root torque introduced with a reverse curve in the archwire to control the labial inclination of the lower incisors.

Fig. 2.148

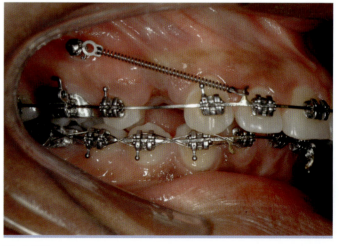

Figs 2.150, 2.151 & 2.152
Frontal and lateral views after the extraction of the upper first premolars. Retraction has been initiated using Nitinol springs from the miniscrews to the hooks welded onto the .019/.025 rectangular stainless steel archwire. The hook to the mesial of the canine is short in height, which creates the necessary vertical component of force for correction of the deep overbite.

Fig. 2.150

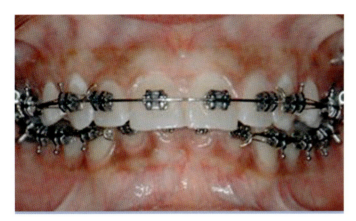

Fig. 2.146

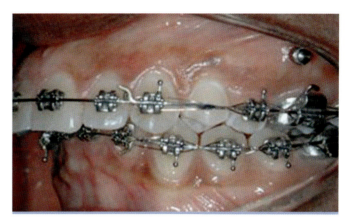

Fig. 2.147

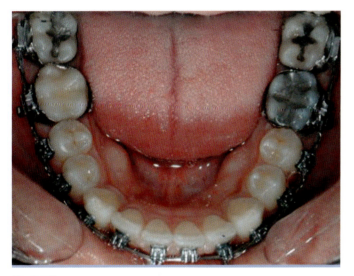

Fig. 2.149

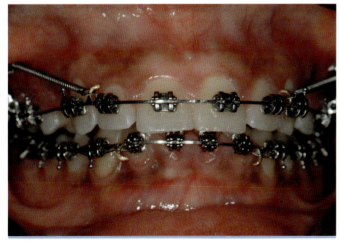

Fig. 2.151

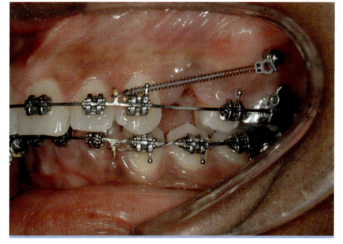

Fig. 2.152

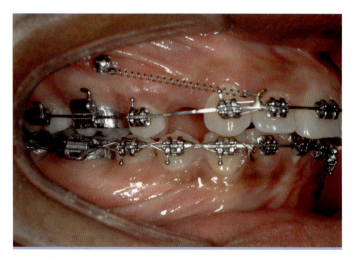

Fig. 2.153

Figs 2.153, 2.154 & 2.155
Frontal and lateral views, 1 month after the application of the space closure mechanics. Overbite correction has started and the absolute anchorage system with miniscrews is in place.

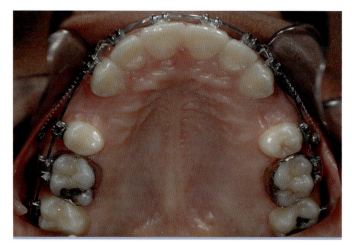

Fig. 2.156

Figs 2.156 & 2.157
Occlusal views of the upper and lower arches at the beginning of the retraction stage. As mentioned above, lower incisor inclination was controlled by labial root torque added to the rectangular archwire.

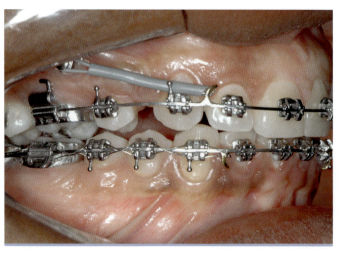

Fig. 2.158

Figs 2.158, 2.159 & 2.160
Lateral and frontal views showing the second retraction system consisting of a ligature wire and elastic modules and a wire protector. At this stage of treatment, the deep overbite was corrected and the upper incisor proclination reduced. There was Class II overcorrection due to spontaneous anterior movement of the mandible.

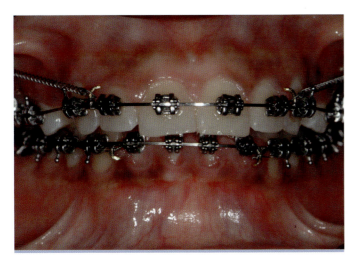

Fig. 2.154

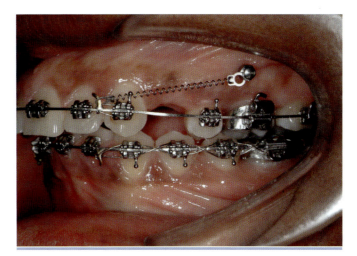

Fig. 2.155

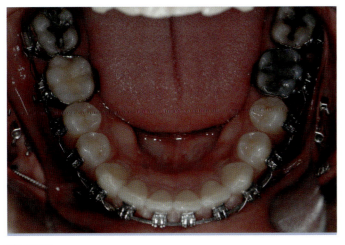

Fig. 2.157

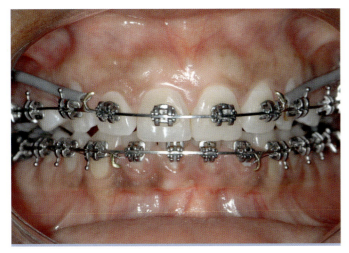

Fig. 2.159

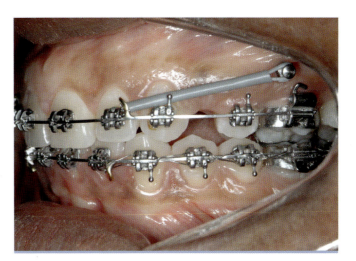

Fig. 2.160

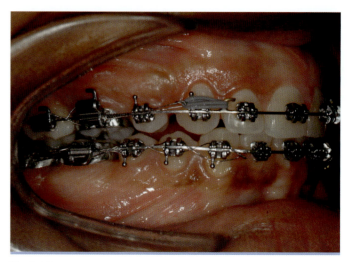

Figs 2.161, 2.162 & 2.163
Frontal and lateral views after removal of the miniscrews. There are buccal tubes on the second molars and a figure-of-eight ligature to prevent space opening. An .018 round stainless steel archwire has been engaged in the upper arch.

Fig. 2.161

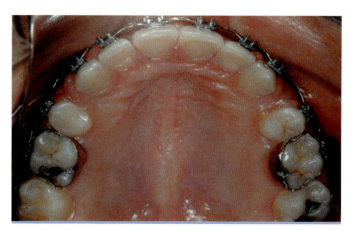

Figs 2.164 & 2.165
Occlusal view of the upper and lower arches with a .018 round stainless steel archwire and molar-to-molar passive laceback in the upper arch to hold the spaces closed. In the lower arch, the .019/.025 rectangular archwire was kept in place.

Fig. 2.164

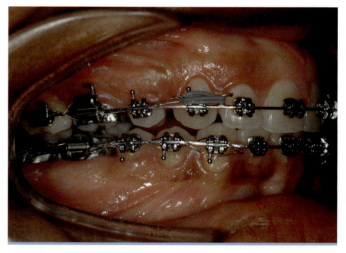

Figs 2.166, 2.167 & 2.168
Frontal and lateral views of a .019/.025 rectangular archwire re-engaged in the upper arch. Palatal root torque was added to the upper incisors, aiming at creating some overjet to allow further retraction of the upper teeth and finish the treatment with the molars in a Class II relationship.

Fig. 2.166

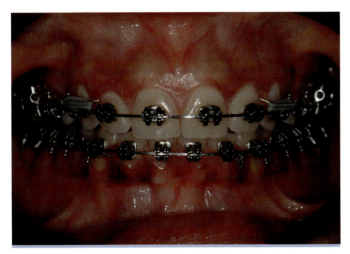

Fig. 2.162

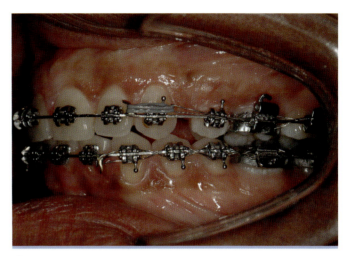

Fig. 2.163

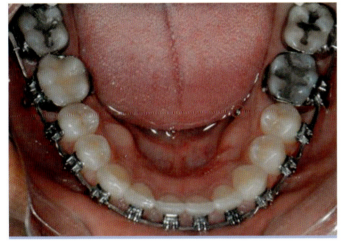

Fig. 2.165

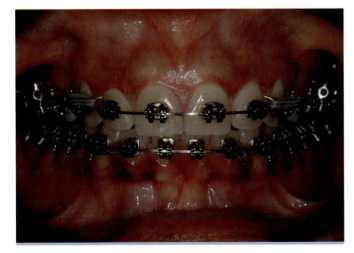

Fig. 2.167

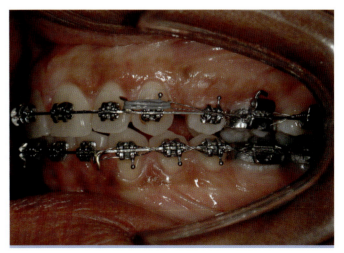

Fig. 2.168

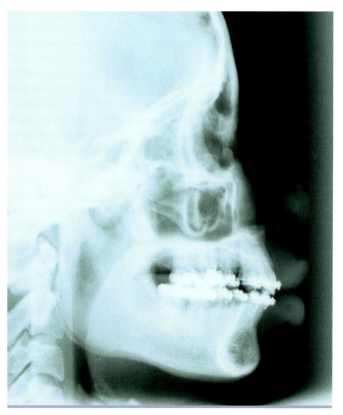

Fig. 2.169

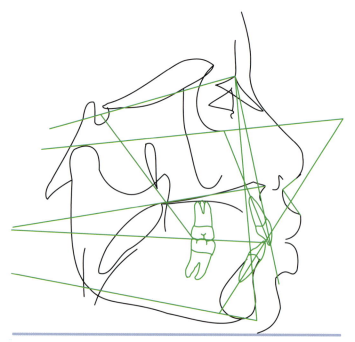

Fig. 2.170

Figs 2.169, 2.170 & 2.171
Interim cephalometric radiograph, tracing and analysis illustrating the need for additional palatal root torque for the upper incisors.

SNA ∠	88º
SNB ∠	80º
ANB ∠	8º
A-N ⊥ FH	7 mm
Po-N ⊥ FH	0 mm
Wits	1 mm
GoGn SN ∠	24º
FH Mx ∠	16º
Mx Md ∠	19º
U1 to A-Po	6 mm
L1 to A-Po	3 mm
U1 to Mx plane ∠	103º
L1 to Md plane ∠	110º
Facial analysis	
Nasolabial ∠	92º
NA ⊥ nose	25 mm
Lip thickness	12.5 mm

Fig. 2.171

Pretreatment ————
Interim ————

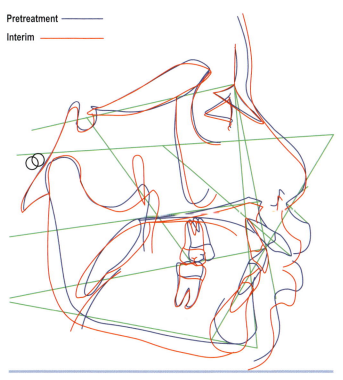

Fig. 2.172

Fig. 2.172

Superimposition of the pretreatment and interim cephalometric tracings. There was a clockwise mandible rotation during the treatment. Point A moved backwards and downwards due to the palatal inclination of the upper incisors.

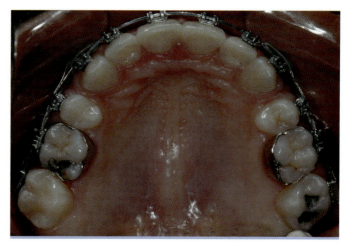

Fig. 2.173

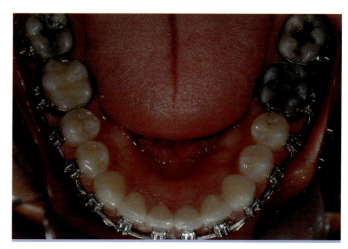

Figs 2.173 & 2.174
Occlusal views of the space closure stage of the extraction sites of the upper first premolars.

Fig. 2.174

Figs 2.176, 2.177 & 2.178
Lateral and frontal views of .019/.025 rectangular stainless steel archwire with palatal root torque for the upper incisors and the retraction system in place, leading to an improvement in the inclination of the incisors. The anchorage system was maintained in place.

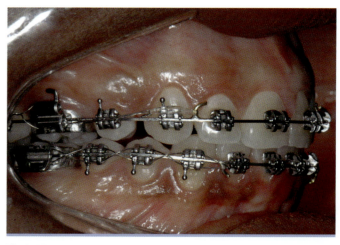

Fig. 2.176

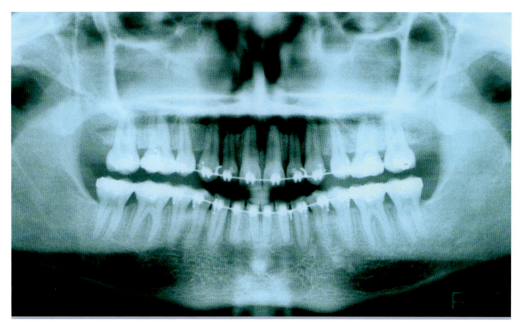

Fig. 2.175

Fig. 2.175
Panoramic radiograph showing achievement of root parallelism.

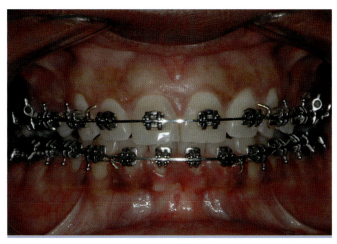

Fig. 2.177

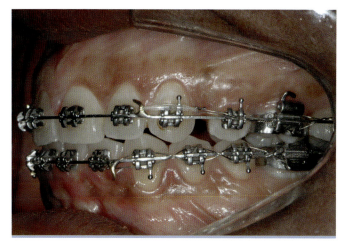

Fig. 2.178

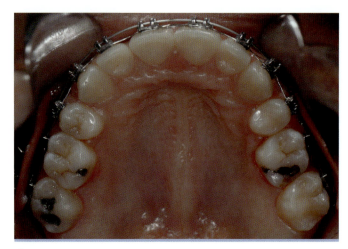

Fig. 2.179

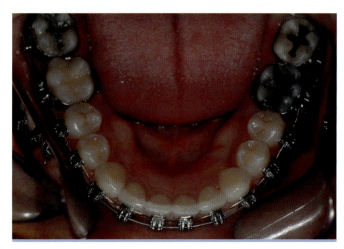

Figs 2.179 & 2.180

Occlusal views illustrating the versatility of the MBT™ Appliance System technique. Lower second molar buccal tubes are being used on the upper first and second molars of the opposite side with a .018 Nitinol archwire. In the lower arch, the .019/.025 rectangular archwire was kept in place.

Fig. 2.180

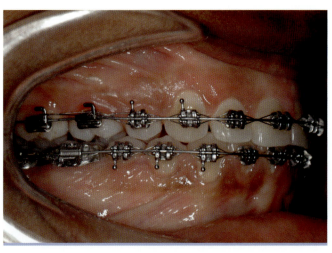

Figs 2.182, 2.183 & 2.184

Illustration of the versatility of the MBT™ Appliance System technique using lower second molar buccal tubes from the opposite side on the upper first and second molars; .018 Nitinol archwires were engaged for re-leveling the dental arches.

Fig. 2.182

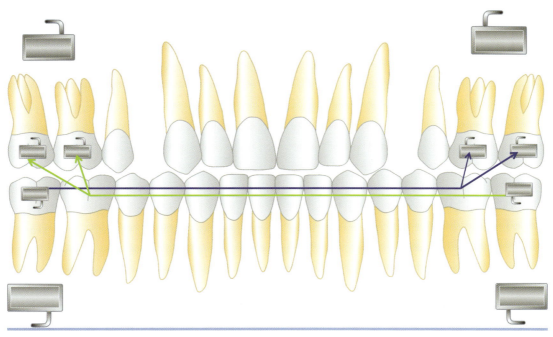

Fig. 2.181

Fig. 2.181
Diagrammatic illustration of the versatility of the MBT™ System Appliance.

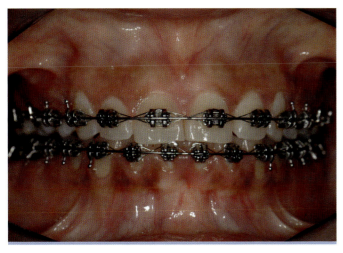

Fig. 2.183

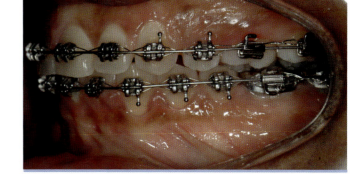

Fig. 2.184

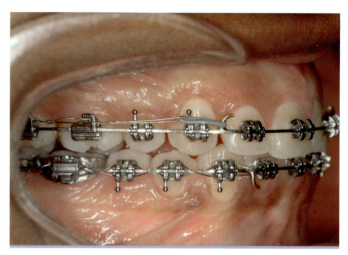

Figs 2.185, 2.186 & 2.187
Frontal and lateral views of the next stage with .019/.025 rectangular stainless steel archwires and the retraction system for final closure of the remaining spaces.

Fig. 2.185

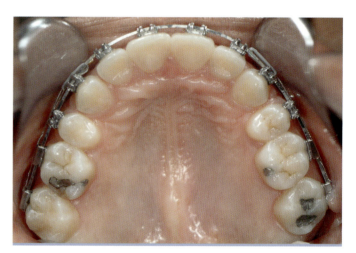

Figs 2.188 & 2.189
Occlusal view of the upper and lower arches with .019/.025 rectangular stainless steel archwires in place. The upper molars do not show rotation, enabling the contact point to be buccal to the first and second molars. Positioning the molars without 10° rotation allows a decrease in the mesiodistal diameter by 2 mm approximately.

Fig. 2.188

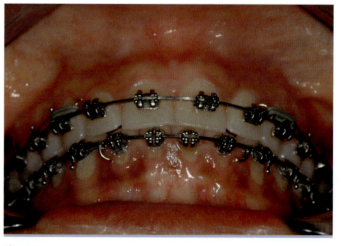

Figs 2.190, 2.191 & 2.192
Figure 2.190 shows the incisor anterior guidance and the lateroprotrusive canine guidance well established after treatment. Figures 2.191 and 2.192 show the leveled curve of Spee.

Fig. 2.190

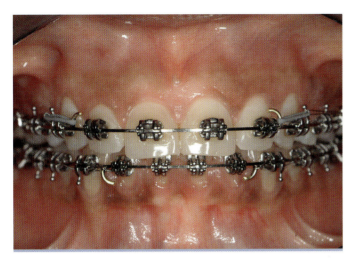

Fig. 2.186

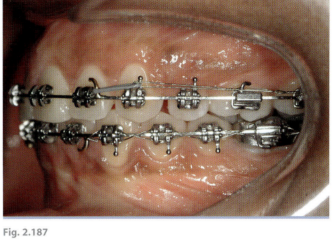

Fig. 2.187

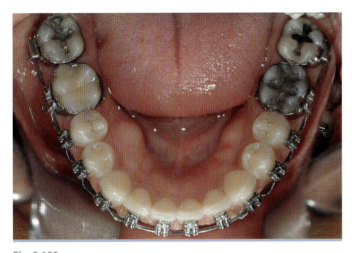

Fig. 2.189

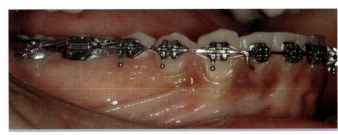

Fig. 2.191

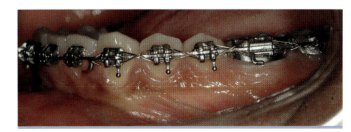

Fig. 2.192

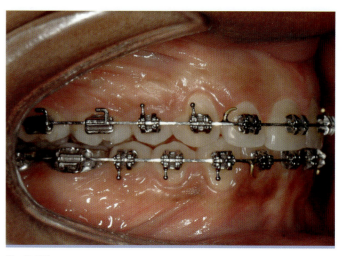

Fig. 2.193

Figs 2.193, 2.194 & 2.195

Continuing final space closure with .019/.025 rectangular stainless steel archwires, still applying MBT™ appliance versatility on the upper molars.

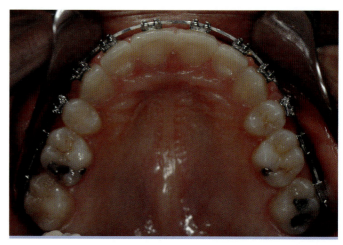

Fig. 2.196

Figs 2.196 & 2.197

Occlusal view after space closure. Arch form and contact points are well established.

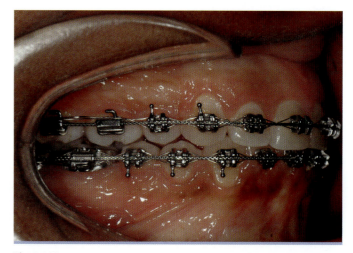

Fig. 2.198

Figs 2.198, 2.199 & 2.200

Settling of the occlusion with .019/.025 rectangular braided archwires. Passive lacebacks with .008 metal ligatures were inserted before engaging the archwire.

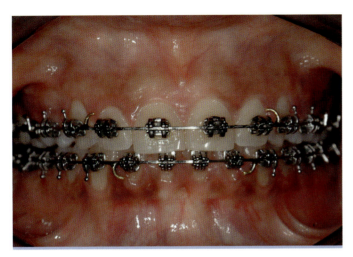

Fig. 2.194

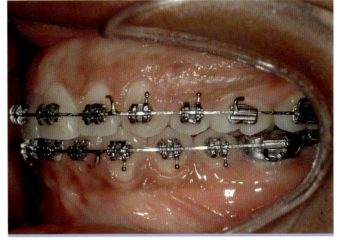

Fig. 2.195

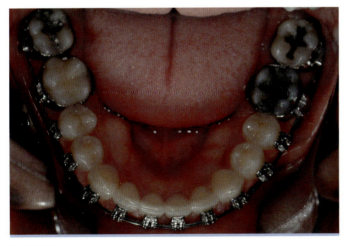

Fig. 2.197

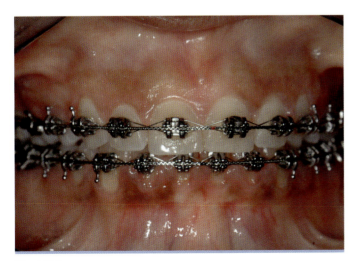

Fig. 2.199

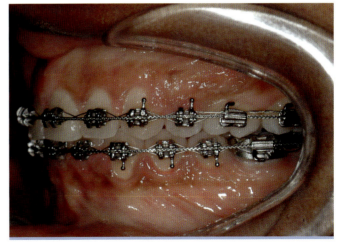

Fig. 2.200

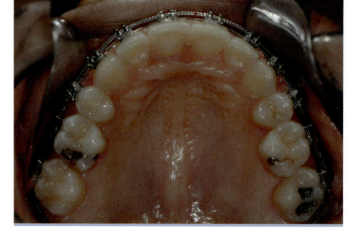

Figs 2.201 & 2.202
Occlusal views of .019/.025 rectangular braided archwires in the upper and lower arches.

Fig. 2.201

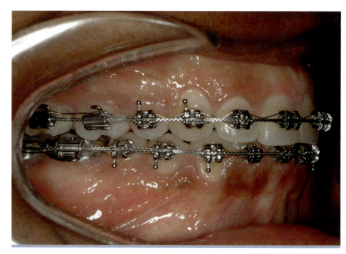

Figs 2.203, 2.204 & 2.205
Triangular 3/16 (4 oz) elastics for final settling of the occlusion, with .019/.025 rectangular braided archwires in place. The .008 ligature passive lacebacks are still in place.

Fig. 2.203

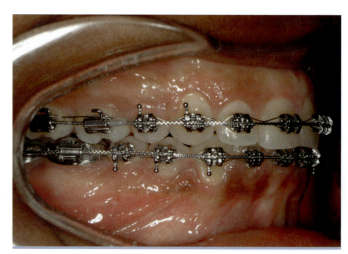

Figs 2.206, 2.207 & 2.208
Frontal and lateral views of the occlusion after 1 month of use of the triangular elastics.

Fig. 2.206

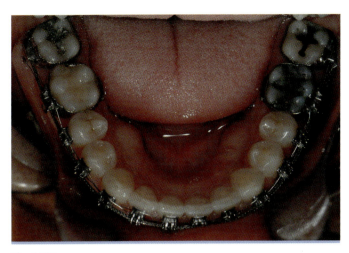

Fig. 2.202

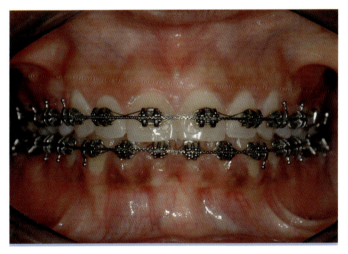

Fig. 2.204

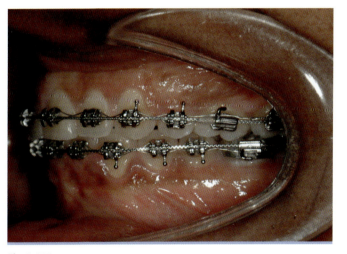

Fig. 2.205

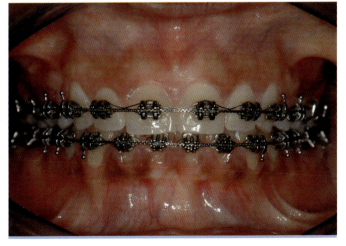

Fig. 2.207

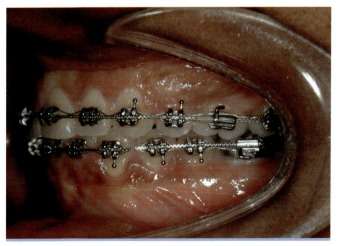

Fig. 2.208

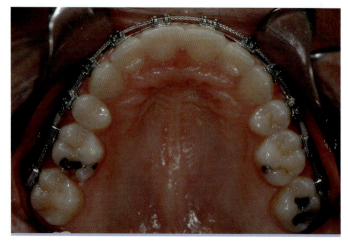

Fig. 2.209

Figs 2.209 & 2.210
Occlusal views at the end of treatment.

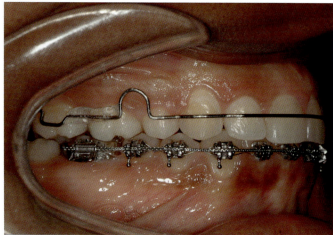

Fig. 2.211

Figs 2.211, 2.212 & 2.213
Fixed appliance removal. First the upper appliance was removed and the Hawley retainer fitted. Then lower second molar bands were removed.

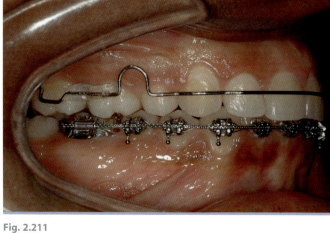

Fig. 2.214

Figs 2.214 & 2.215
Occlusal view after the removal of the fixed appliance from the upper arch and lower second molar bands.

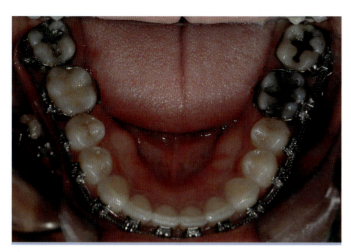

Fig. 2.210

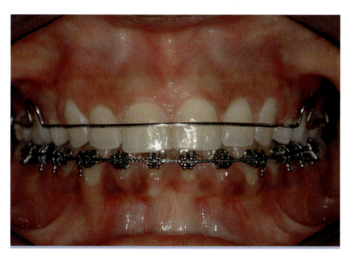

Fig. 2.212

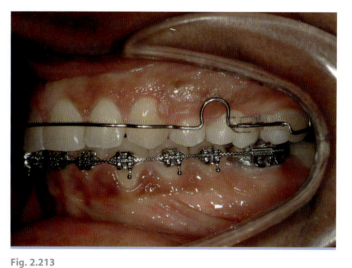

Fig. 2.213

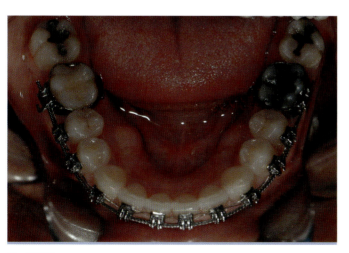

Fig. 2.215

Figs 2.216, 2.217 & 2.218

Lower appliance removal and fixed 3 × 3 retainer placed in the lower arch. A perfect Class II molar relationship and Class I canine relationship is seen. The overbite and centerlines are corrected.

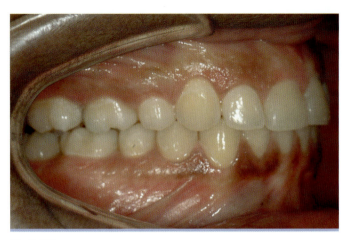

Fig. 2.216

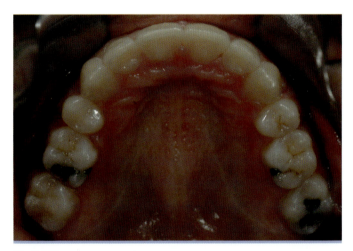

Fig. 2.219

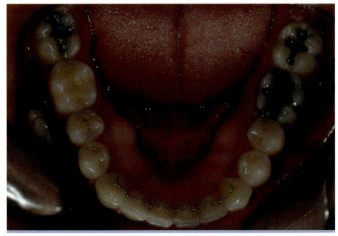

Figs 2.219 & 2.220

Post-treatment occlusal views of the upper and lower arches.

Fig. 2.220

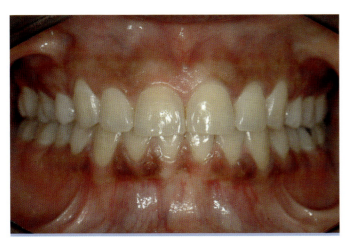

Fig. 2.217

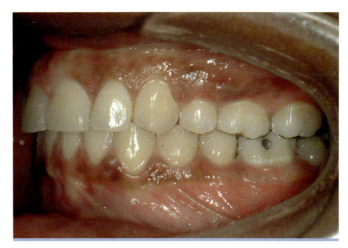

Fig. 2.218

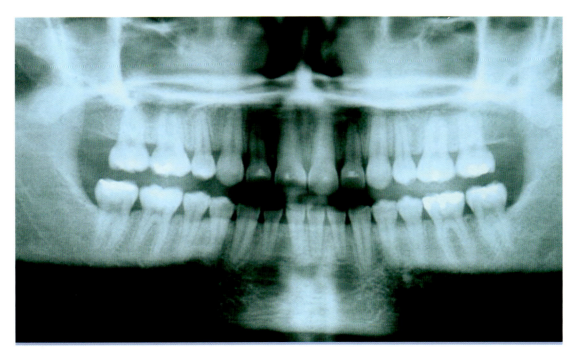

Fig. 2.221

Fig. 2.221
Final panoramic radiograph showing maintenance of root parallelism. The apex of the lower incisor roots are rounded due to the vertical forces applied to correct the deep overbite.

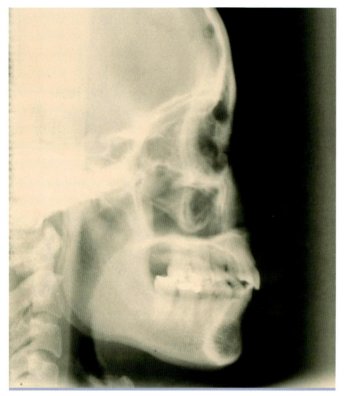

Fig. 2.222

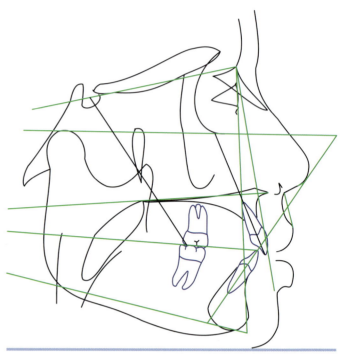

Fig. 2.223

Figs 2.222, 2.223 & 2.224
The final cephalometric radiograph, tracing and analysis showing the incisors to be well positioned in the maxillary and mandibular osseous bases.

Figs 2.226 & 2.227
Post-treatment extraoral photographs showing good facial symmetry and lip seal.

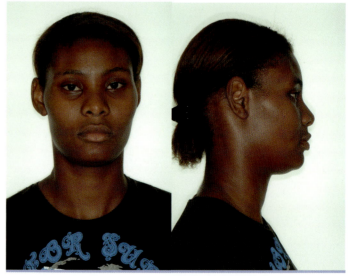

Fig. 2.226   Fig. 2.227

Development of the second and third molars

The upper second molar is the seventh tooth in each quadrant of the upper and lower dental arches, and is similar to the first molar morphologically, although smaller in size. When describing this tooth, a direct comparison should be made with the first molars, regarding its function and development. In 1935, Schwartz[3] evaluated the size of the second molar crown and found the height of the crown varied from 5.7 mm to 8.3 mm. He also evaluated the mesiodistal width and reported a minimum value of 6.5 mm and a maximum value of 10.5 mm.

The second molar is also the seventh tooth to erupt, and this normally occurs after the eruption of the second premolars, when a person is 11–13 years of age, depending on their gender. However, the lower second molars usually erupt before the upper ones, within a period of a few months to half a year (Figs 3.2, 3.3 & 3.4). Another important point to consider is the space available to accommodate the second molar.

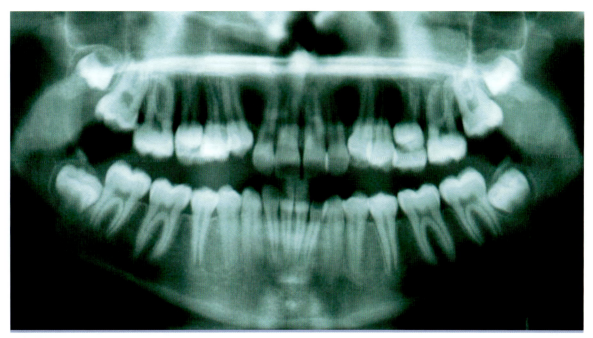

Fig. 3.2

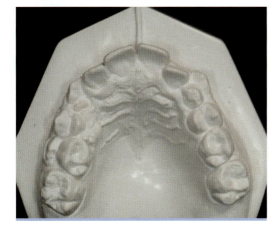

Fig. 3.3

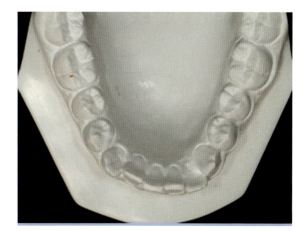

Fig. 3.4

Figs 3.2, 3.3 & 3.4 Panoramic radiograph and study models showing that the lower second molars usually erupt before the upper second molars.

The upper third molars are considered to be the most variable teeth in the dental arch. Their average mesiodistal width varies from 6.5 mm to 11.5 mm. In 1976, Della Serra[4] reported that the upper third molar crowns presented with different shapes, varying from the typical molar shape to much more conical and simpler shapes. To reiterate, this tooth is frequently smaller in size, with a more simple shape. Third molar crowns are also frequently buccally oriented and distally angulated. Due to their anatomical and positional variability, it is critical to carefully select cases that will undergo second molar extraction. The shape and the size of third molars is decisive for the success of treatment.

At the beginning of their formation, upper third molar crowns are angulated distally (Fig. 3.5). However, this tendency decreases as the maxillary tuberosity grows. If there is no growth, third molar impaction is highly likely. If first and second molars are distalized while the third molar is developing, tooth impaction may occur due to the decrease in space in the posterior segment of the dental arch.

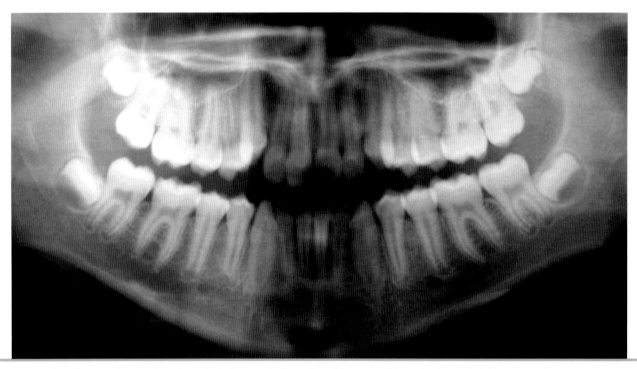

Fig. 3.5 Panoramic radiograph showing that, due to lack of space, the formation of the upper third molars is usually initiated with the crown distally tipped.

The occlusal surface of the lower third molars is often slightly tipped mesiolingually during the initial calcification period. Space for their eruption is linked to mandibular growth and remodeling of the mandibular ramus, that is, bone is resorbed on the anterior surface of the ramus and deposited on its posterior surface, thus increasing the length of the mandibular body and the space available for teeth to erupt in.

Lower third molar eruption is unpredictable, and even if space is available, their satisfactory eruption is not guaranteed. Third molar impaction occurs not only due to a lack of space in the posterior segment of the dental arch, but also due to unfavorable tooth inclination. The best method of avoiding third molar impaction is extraction of the second molars. Such extractions are therefore indicated when the third molar roots are developing (Fig. 3.6).

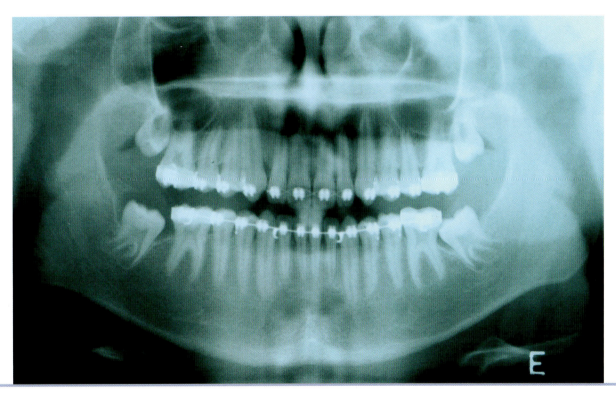

Fig. 3.6 Panoramic radiograph showing how space created by second molar extraction has allowed distalization of the first molar and space for the eruption of the developing third molars.

Why should second molars be extracted?

A large proportion of the routine work of an orthodontist is treating sagittal Class II malocclusions, which is the most common malocclusion among patients seeking orthodontic treatment. Class II malocclusions are frequently accompanied by compromised facial esthetics, which is best dealt with in the mixed dentition. However, patients do not always seek treatment in the mixed dentition. Rather, they postpone treatment to adolescence, a period which is often associated with poor patient cooperation. In such adolescent cases, second molar extractions offers a valid alternative treatment option for Class II treatment.[1]

As mentioned in the introduction, the main goals of a second molar extraction treatment are preventing third molar impaction (Fig. 3.7) and

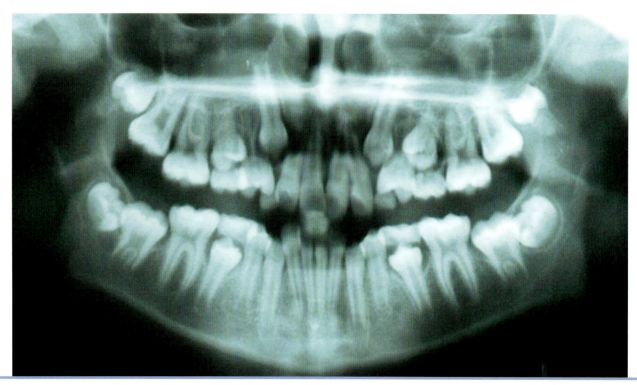

Fig. 3.7 Panoramic radiograph showing inadequate space for the eruption of the second and the third molars.

making first molar uprighting easier. These extractions create some space distal to the archwire, isolating the third molar from the remaining teeth, enabling its anterocclusal movement and its eruption in contact with the distalized first molar (Figs 3.8, 3.9, 3.10, 3.11 & 3.12). A third molar of good shape and size is an ideal substitute for second molars.

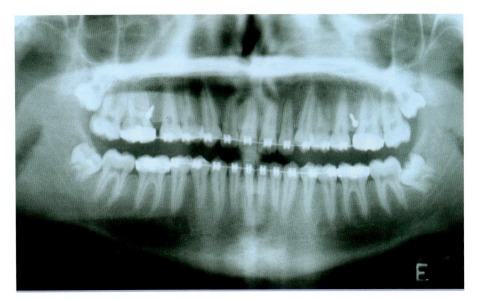

Fig. 3.8

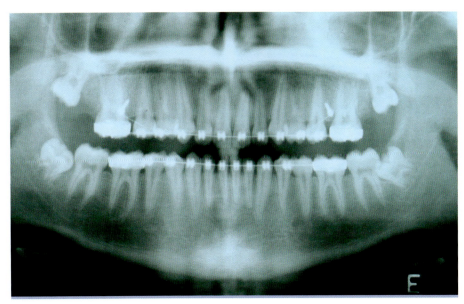

Fig. 3.9

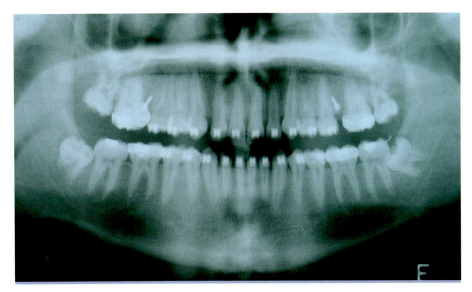

Figs 3.8, 3.9 & 3.10 Panoramic radiograph of a patient who underwent orthodontic treatment with upper second molar extractions. The spaces created enabled optimal eruption of the third molars.

Fig. 3.10

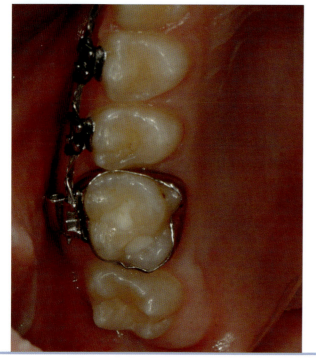

Fig. 3.11

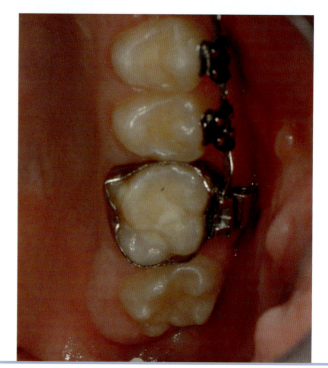

Fig. 3.12

Figs 3.11 & 3.12 Occlusal view at the end of the corrective treatment with the third molars fully erupted, showing perfect alignment and establishment of the contact points with the first molars.

Currently, there are effective devices available to distalize first molars. However, significant distalization of first molars may cause third molar impaction and lead to tooth extraction in a few cases. Therefore, if one of the molars has to be extracted, why not extract the second molar? This approach allows easier movement of the first molar and decreases treatment time.

Another important consideration is the establishment of the contact points. These should be present at the end of treatment, as the tooth extracted is the posterior-most rather than from within the arch.

When observing the dental arches in second molar extraction cases, there is no clinical sign of tooth extraction. This is due to the third molar erupting straight into contact with the first molar.

When second molars are extracted, treatment is generally finished with 28 teeth in situ. Therefore, again in a patient with premolar and molar crowding, second molar extraction is a good treatment option. Such a procedure establishes enough space for correction of crowding (Figs 3.13, 3.14, 3.15, 3.16 & 3.17) and avoids third molar impaction.

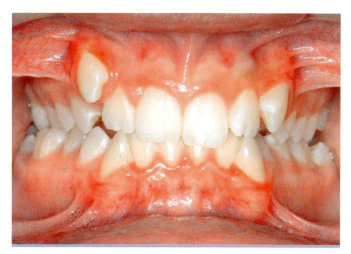

Fig. 3.13

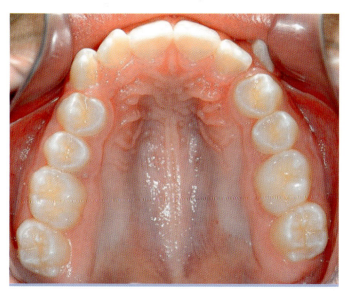

Fig. 3.14

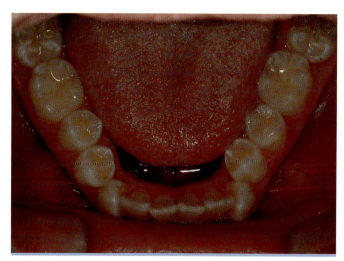

Fig. 3.15

Figs 3.13, 3.14 & 3.15 Occlusal and frontal views of the upper and lower dental arches before upper and lower second molar extractions and the start of orthodontic treatment to move the first molars distally.

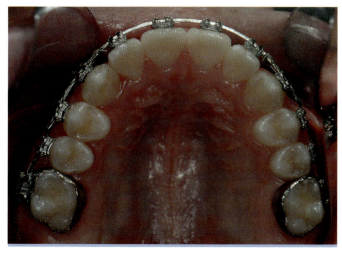

Fig. 3.16

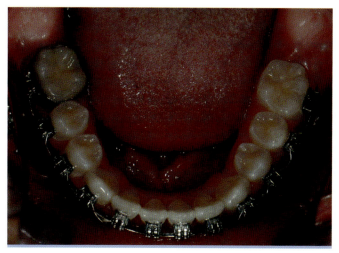

Fig. 3.17

Figs 3.16 & 3.17 Occlusal views at the end of the corrective treatment showing perfect alignment and contact points before the eruption of the third molars. The appliance was removed at this stage, while waiting for the eruption of the third molars.

However, it is to be remembered that second molar extractions cannot replace premolar extractions. The indications for each are entirely different. In summary:[4,5]

- Second molar extractions are indicated for patients presenting with Class II or Class III malocclusions in whom the aim is to make first molar distalization easier.
- Premolar extractions are indicated in patients presenting with a vertical growth pattern, significant anterior crowding, incisor proclination and lack of lip competence.

When should second molars be extracted?

Before extracting a second molar, it is necessary to evaluate the shape and the mesiodistal height of its crown, as well as the state of development of the third molar tooth germ. A panoramic radiograph should be taken to check the posterior segments of the dental arches, as it allows satisfactory assessment of third molar size, the amount of root calcification and the relationship between the tooth germ and the second molar root.[6] If the radiograph image is blurred, and it is difficult to visualize the size of the third molar germ,

it is necessary to take a periapical radiograph. The shape of the third molar is decisive for the treatment plan.

As mentioned briefly in the introduction, the best time to extract second molars is when the crown of the third molar is completely formed and the roots have achieved one-third of their development.[7] Thus, the tooth germ of the third molar will move anteriorly, erupting in the space of the second molar and in contact with the distalized first molar (see Fig. 3.1). In over 90% of the cases, third molars erupt in a good or in an acceptable condition after the extraction of the second molars.[7] Some upper third molars may erupt in crossbite, and should this occur, it will be necessary to use an orthodontic appliance to correct the bite.

When second molar extraction is carried out in a patient with late maturation of the third molars, the treatment is finished before the third molars erupt. The teeth may take 2 years to erupt after the treatment. Therefore the appliance removal protocol should be to remove the appliance in the lower arch, but keeping the tubes on the molars. This protocol is followed to prevent the extrusion of the lower second molars, which have no antagonist teeth during that period of time (Figs 3.18 & 3.19).

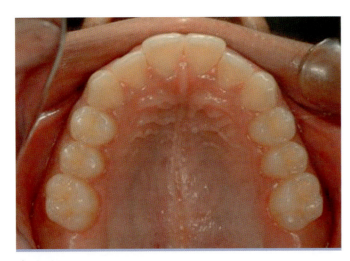

Fig. 3.18

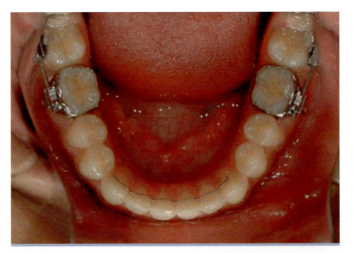

Fig. 3.19

Figs 3.18 & 3.19 Upper bands on the first molars and bonded tubes on the second molars kept in situ while waiting for the eruption of the third molars.

Characteristics of patients who undergo second molar extractions

Second molar extraction is one of the treatment options for Class II malocclusions in adolescent patients. It should not be forgotten that the orthodontic diagnosis is based on morphological characteristics and that careful selection of patients who will undergo such extractions is important so that these extractions do not compromise the final occlusion. This requires awareness of some characteristics presented by these patients.

Graber[8] reported that upper second molar extractions would speed up the treatment of Angle Class II division 1 malocclusions. He also described some characteristics that should be observed before submitting a patient to second molar extractions:

• Reduced overbite
• Excessive labial inclination of the upper incisors
• Third molars in place, showing good shape and size.

Currently, orthodontic treatment is customized according to the facial characteristics of the patient, including certain aspects of the muscle pattern. Second molar extractions are best indicated in patients with mild meso- and dolichofacial patterns, who are the great majority of patients undergoing dental extractions.[9] Patients with a horizontal growth pattern and deep overbite are not suitable for second molar extractions, as the dentoalveolar effect of the mechanics applied will result in a clockwise rotation of the occlusal plane,[10] thus increasing the already deep overbite. In these cases, some clinical maneuvers are needed to avoid these undesired effects, such as adding reverse curve to the lower archwire.

Another characteristic that should be noted is the stability of the lower dental arch. There should be no or mild crowding in the anterior segment, with the incisors well positioned, as severe crowding and/or increased incisor proclination require premolars extractions to harmonize the lower arch. Therefore for these cases, second molar extractions are not indicated.

Considering the interarch relationship, second molar extractions are indicated in patients with severe Class II malocclusions (over 50% of patients). In patients with minor sagittal discrepancies, conventional treatment options should be used to distalize the first molars.

In summary, the following characteristics of patients are suitable for second molar extractions:

• Adolescent age
• Mild meso- or dolichofacial facial pattern
• Third molars in place, with good shape and size
• Severe Class II interarch relationship
• Stable lower dental arch (with only mild arch length discrepancy).

Management of the distalizing mechanics

Andrews,[11] when developing the Straight-Wire appliance, noted among his findings the mesial angulation of tooth crowns. The whole dentition undergoes anteroposterior movement, caused by the action of the masticatory muscles, that is, the mesial movement of teeth is physiological. Hence when distalization is indicated, the movement in the distal direction is anti-physiologic and difficult to achieve. The recommendation to extract the second or the third molars to create space in the posterior segment of the dental arches and to facilitate easier distalization of the first molars was discussed above.[12] The treatment mechanics are customized for each patient and the distalizing device used depends on the facial pattern as well as on the orthodontist's preference. There are a great variety of devices on the market that can be used to distalize the upper first molars, such as headgear, Class II elastics with sliding jigs and orthodontic miniscrews (Figs 3.20, 3.21 & 3.22).

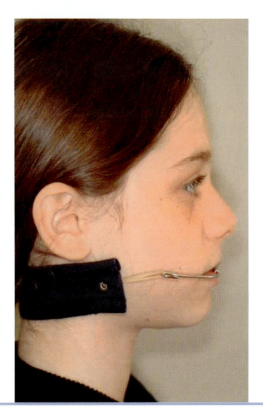

Fig. 3.20

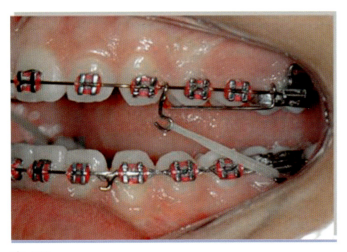

Fig. 3.21

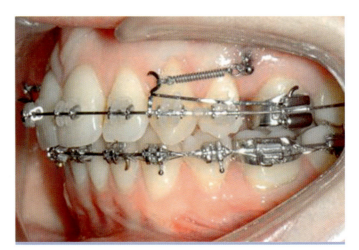

Fig. 3.22

Figs 3.20, 3.21 & 3.22 Distalization of the upper first molars with headgear and Class II elastics with the distalizing jig. Figure 3.22 shows a miniscrew inserted to the mesial of the molar and being used in association with a sliding jig.

After the extraction of the second molars the distalization of the upper first molars is a very easy procedure, as there is decompression of the posterior segment of the dental arch, with adequate space for the distalization of the upper first molar, and, at the same time, impaction of the third molars is avoided. Treatment time decreases considerably due to quicker establishment of the Class I interarch relationship.

Eruption of third molars after second molar extraction

As shown by clinical experience, third molars erupt satisfactorily in the vast majority of second molar extraction cases. When second molar extractions are carried out before the formation of the roots of the third molars, the eruption of these teeth is accelerated and frequently occurs by the end of the orthodontic treatment, when the fixed appliances are still in place. If the second molars are extracted when the third molars are late in maturing, the appliances should be removed when the remaining treatment goals have been achieved, even if the third molars are yet to erupt (Figs 3.23 & 3.24, 3.25, 3.26, 3.27, 3.28).

Although, as mentioned already, upper third molars erupt in good or acceptable condition in over 90% of second molar extraction cases, some may erupt in a crossbite. If this occurs, it is necessary to place tubes on the molars to correct the crossbite.[2,13]

Another point to note is the remaining root formation of the third molars after the extraction of the second molars. The third molars are known to display anatomic variability with the roots frequently tipped due to a lack of space in the posterior segment of the dental arch. With the extraction of the second molars to create space in the posterior segment of the dental arch, the chances of good root formation of the third molars are improved.

Cavanaugh[14] carried out clinical and radiographic evaluation of eruption of the third molars after the extraction of the second molars in 25 subjects. He reported no impactions of the third molars, very low incidence of fused roots and an improvement in the mesiodistal angulation of the third molar roots. He concluded that these extractions, when carried out in carefully selected patients, are the best treatment option in many situations, as it is a reliable and conservative procedure.

In 2007, Zanelato[15] studied on study models the position of third molars that had erupted spontaneously in cases treated with second molar extraction and compared this with the position of the third molars in a sample of subjects presenting with normal natural occlusions. The author reported that the third molars, when substituting for the second molars, show good mesiodistal and buccolingual root positions. The size of the clinical crowns of the third molars were acceptable in both the male and the female subjects. No significant difference in clinical crown height was observed between the groups.

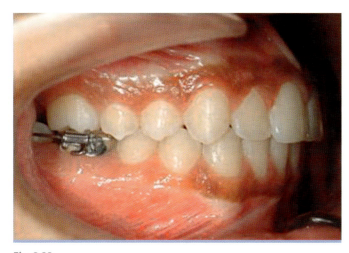

Fig. 3.23

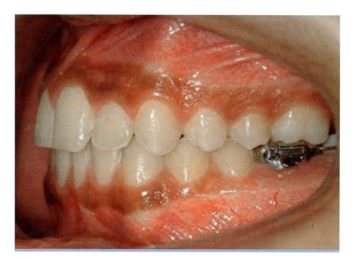

Fig. 3.24

Figs 3.23 and 3.24 Lateral views of the end of the corrective orthodontic treatment, before the eruption of the upper third molars. The lower appliance was kept in place on the first and the second molars until the eruption of the third molars.

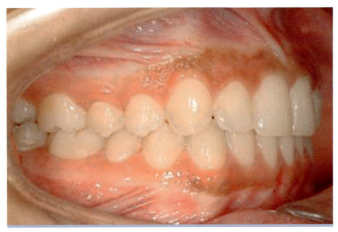

Fig. 3.25

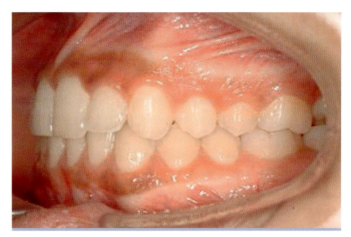

Fig. 3.26

Figs 3.25 and 3.26 Lateral views 5 years after removal of fixed appliances. The interarch relationship is stable with a good premolar and canine intercuspation, corrected centerlines and stable overjet and overbite.

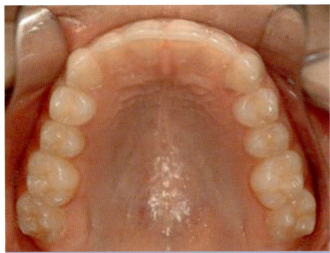

Fig. 3.27

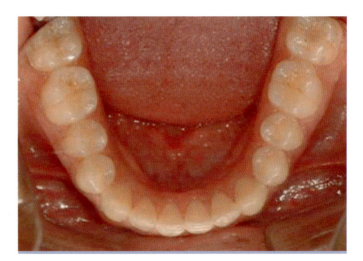

Fig. 3.28

Figs 3.27 and 3.28 Occlusal views 5 years after the appliance was removed and also the fixed 3 × 3 retainer. Note the good dental arch forms with 28 teeth and well-established contact points.

References

1. Zanelato R C, Trevisi H J, Zanelato A C T 2000 Extração dos segundos molares superiores: uma nova abordagem para tratamentos da Classe I I, em pacientes adolescentes. Revista Dental Press de Ortodontia e Ortopedia Facial 5:64–75

2. Richardson M E, Richardson A 1993 Lower third molar development subsequent to second molar extraction. American Journal of Orthodontics and Dentofacial Orthopedics 104:566–574

3. Schwartz J R 1935 Practical dental: anatomy and tooth carving. Dental Items of Interest, Henry Kimpton's Medical Publishing House, New York

4. Della Serra O 1976 Anatomia dental, 2nd ed. Artes Médicas, São Paulo, p 318

5. Bennett J C, McLaughlin R P 1998 O tratamento ortodôntico da dentição com aparelho pré-ajustado. Artes Médicas, São Paulo

6. Janson G 2002 Influência do padrão facial na decisão de extrações. Revista Dental Press de Ortodontia e Ortopedia Facial 7:41–47

7. Rosé M M, Verdon P 1983 Ortodoncia de Mollin: técnica e interpretacíon filosófica. Adrogué Gráfica, Buenos Aires

8. Graber T M 1969 Maxillary second molar extractions in Class II malocclusion. American Journal of Orthodontics and Dentofacial Orthopedics 56:331–353

9. Crepaldi A 1999 Avaliação das medidas cefalométricas verticais, padrão Trevisi, dos pacientes tratados com extração dos segundos molares superiores permanentes. Trabalho de Conclusão de Curso (Especialização em Ortodontia), Universidade de Cuiabá

10. Woelfel J B, Scheid R C 2000 Anatomia dental: sua relevância para a Odontologia, 5th ed. Guanabara Koogan, Rio de Janeiro, p 151

11. Andrews L F 1989 Straight wire: the concept and appliance. L A Wells, San Diego

12. Zanelato R C 2003 Entrevista. Revista Dental Press de Ortodontia e Ortopedia Facial 2:5–8

13. Richardson M E 1998 O terceiro molar: uma perspectiva ortodôntica. Revista Dental Press de Ortodontia e Ortopedia Facial 3:103–117

14. Cavanaugh J J 1985 Third molar changes following second molar extractions. Angle Orthodontist 55:70–76

15. Zanelato R C 2007 Evaluación de las coronas de los primeros e terceros molares superiores. Revista Española de Ortodoncia 37:79–101

CHAPTER 3 CLINICAL CASE 1

Name: CCC
Sex: Female
Age: 15 years, 8 months
Facial pattern: Brachyfacial
Skeletal pattern: Class III

Diagnosis

Dental and skeletal Class III malocclusion, bilateral posterior crossbite, anterior crossbite, upper anterior crowding with blocked out upper left canine and upper centerline deviation to the left side.

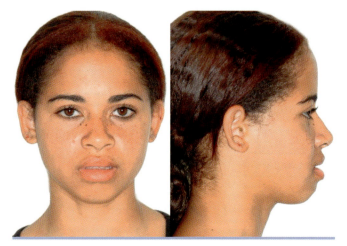

Fig. 3.29   Fig. 3.30

Orthodontic treatment plan

Upper and lower second molar extractions, upper arch expansion, lower molar distalization, correction of the interarch relationship, decrowding and alignment of the anterior teeth with correction of upper centerline and the anterior crossbite.

Figs 3.29 & 3.30
Pretreatment extraoral photographs showing facial symmetry and lip incompetence; the lateral view shows the Class III skeletal pattern.

Appliances used in the treatment

- Lip bumper in the lower arch
- SmartClip™ Self-Ligating Appliance in both upper and lower dental arches

- Class III elastics
- Vertical elastics for posterior crossbite correction
- Hawley retainer in the upper arch
- 3 × 3 fixed retainer in the lower arch

Case report

The treatment plan included upper and lower second molar extractions to gain space, correct the upper crowding, achieve a Class I molar relationship and provide good vertical and horizontal control of the teeth during orthodontic biomechanics.

The second molars were extracted and the lip bumper was placed in the lower arch to initiate molar distalization. The SmartClip™ Self-Ligating Appliance was placed in the upper dental arch and a .014 round Nitinol superelastic archwire was engaged to initiate arch expansion and alignment. Next, a .014 round stainless steel archwire with an omega loop was engaged on the upper arch to continue decrowding and alignment of the anterior teeth and to increase the dental arch length.

After alignment of the anterior teeth, an open coil spring with a .016 round Nitinol archwire was engaged to open space for the upper left canine and correct the upper centerline. The aligning and the leveling of the lower dental arch were carried out with .014 and .016 round Nitinol superelastic archwires.

After creation of the necessary space for the upper left canine, a .014 round Nitinol superelastic archwire was engaged again for further alignment. At this stage of treatment, 3/16 (4 oz) vertical elastics were also used to correct the molar crossbite.

Final leveling was done with .017/.025 and .019/.025 rectangular Nitinol archwires. During this stage of treatment, the patient continued to use the lip bumper to maintain the anchorage in the lower posterior segments. The distalization of the upper first molars was achieved simply with the extraction of the second molars and the forces generated by the SmartClip™ Self-Ligating Appliance.

Space closure was carried out on .019/.025 rectangular stainless steel archwires, with prewelded hooks to the mesial of the canines, using .009 metal ligatures connected to elastic modules. Class III 5/16 (4 oz) elastics were used to correct the molar relationship and the overjet of the anterior teeth. After closure of the spaces, a .009 passive tieback was placed from the molars to the hooks prewelded to the mesial of the canines. They were kept in place until the occlusion had stabilized. In the final stage of treatment, a braided archwire was engaged in the upper arch and 3/16 (4 oz) triangular elastics were placed to settle the occlusion.

The fixed appliances were removed after achieving perfect intercuspation of the teeth and optimization of the functional movements. At this stage of treatment, the lower right third molar erupted in contact with the distal of the lower right first molar. Retention involved a Hawley retainer on the upper arch and a fixed 3 × 3 retainer in the lower arch.

Post-treatment follow-up included taking panoramic radiographs to check the eruption of the remaining third molars. It was verified that these teeth erupted in contact with the first molars. There was no need for further treatment to align and upright these teeth. The final result achieved the functional and esthetic goals of treatment. The patient was very pleased with this final result.

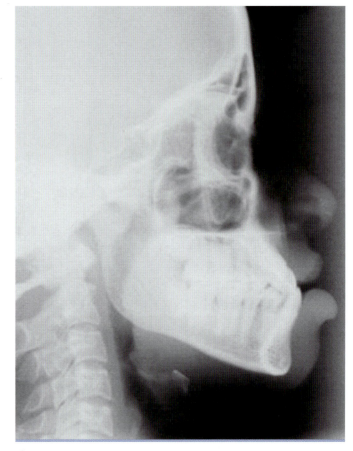

Figs 3.31, 3.32 & 3.33
Cephalometric radiograph, tracing and analysis showing the Class III skeletal pattern, with a Wits of −5 mm and vertical measurements within the normal range.

Fig. 3.31

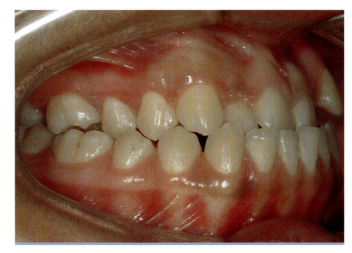

Figs 3.34, 3.35 & 3.36
Pretreatment intraoral photographs showing hypoplastic maxilla, Class III molar relationship, bilateral posterior crossbite, anterior crossbite, upper centreline deviation and blocked out upper left canine.

Fig. 3.34

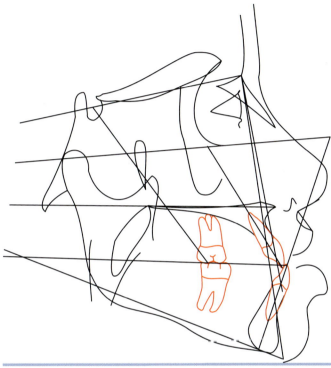

Fig. 3.32

SNA ∠	89º
SNB ∠	87º
ANB ∠	2º
A-N ⊥ FH	7 mm
Po-N ⊥ FH	7 mm
Wits	–5 mm
GoGn SN ∠	32º
FH Md ∠	25º
Mx Md ∠	20º
U1 to A-Po	4 mm
L1 to A-Po	6 mm
U1 to Mx plane ∠	123º
L1 to Md plane ∠	88º
Facial analysis	
Nasolabial ∠	80º
NA ⊥ nose	27 mm
Lip thickness	13 mm

Fig. 3.33

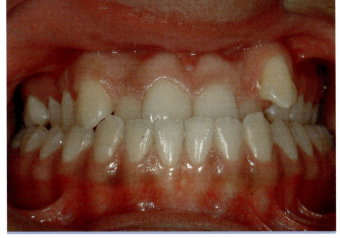

Fig. 3.35

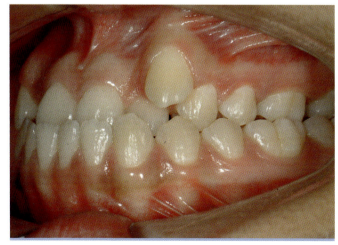

Fig. 3.36

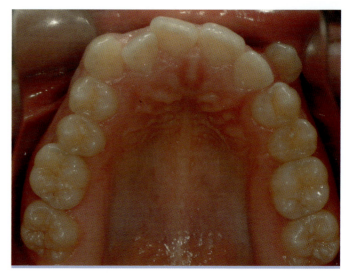

Fig. 3.37

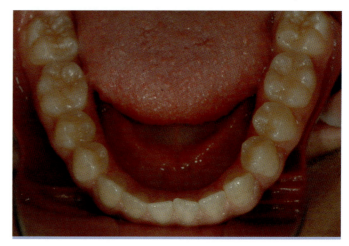

Figs 3.37 & 3.38
Occlusal views showing the severity of the upper anterior crowding and the blocked out left upper canine. The lower dental arch is well aligned with normally inclined incisors.

Fig. 3.38

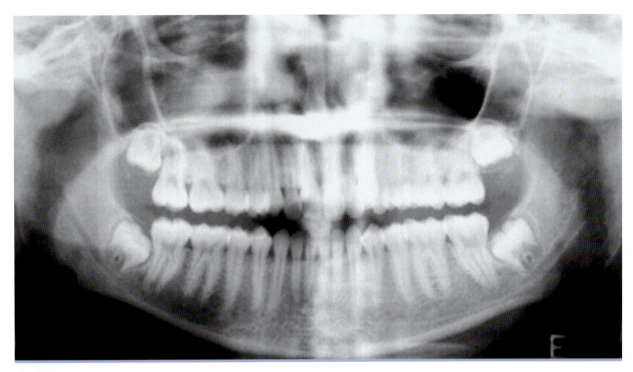

Fig. 3.39

Fig. 3.39
Panoramic radiograph showing the third molars of good size and shape and calcification of the initial third of the root.

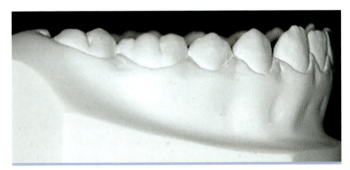

Fig. 3.40

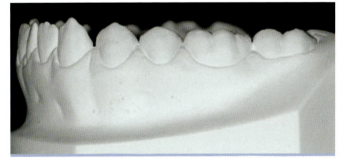

Fig. 3.41

Figs 3.40 & 3.41
Lateral views of the lower arch on the study models showing a flat curve of Spee.

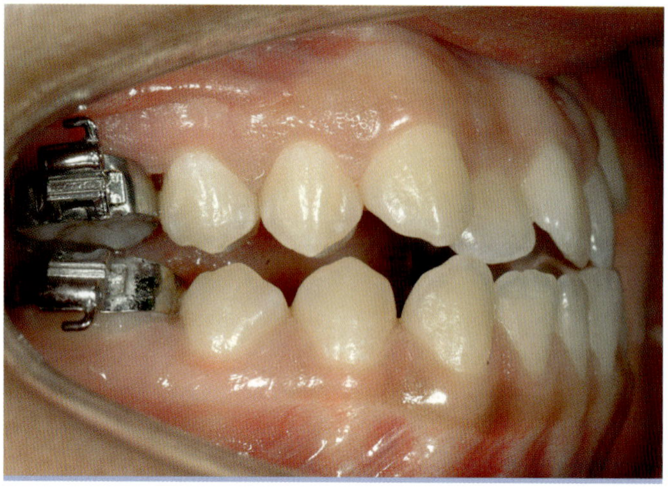

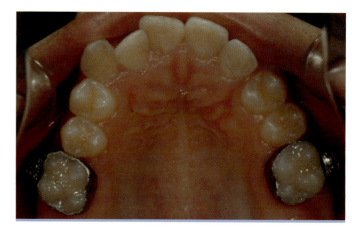

Fig. 3.42

Figs 3.42, 3.43 & 3.44

Frontal and lateral views of bands with double buccal tubes on the first molars for the lip bumper.

Fig. 3.45

Figs 3.45 & 3.46

Occlusal views of the upper and lower dental arches. The bands were placed after the extraction of the second molars.

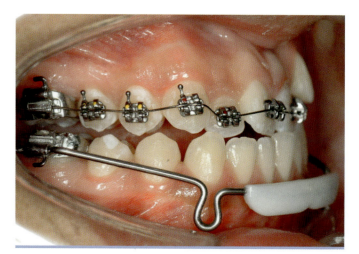

Fig. 3.47

Figs 3.47, 3.48 & 3.49

Frontal and lateral views of the SmartClip™ Self-ligating Appliance in the upper arch with a .014 round Nitinol superelastic archwire initiating the alignment. The lip bumper is in place in the lower arch, enabling distal movement of the lower first molars.

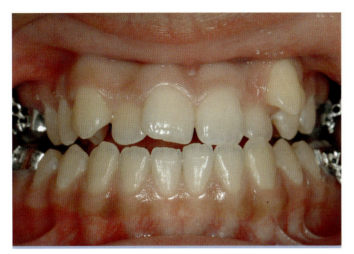

Fig. 3.43

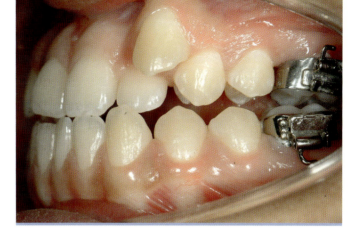

Fig. 3.44

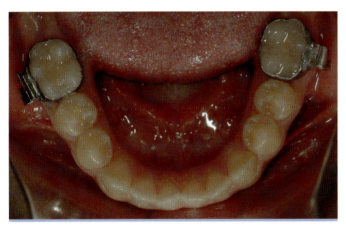

Fig. 3.46

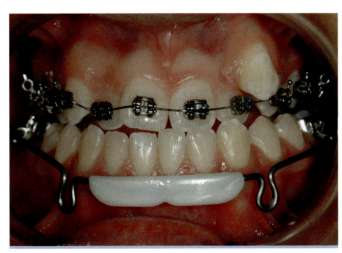

Fig. 3.48

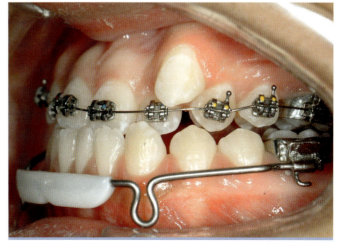

Fig. 3.49

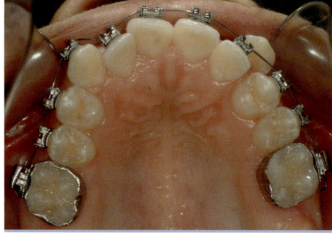

Figs 3.50 & 3.51
Occlusal views showing the SmartClip™ Self-Ligating Appliance System, .014 round archwire in the upper arch and the lip bumper in the lower arch.

Fig. 3.50

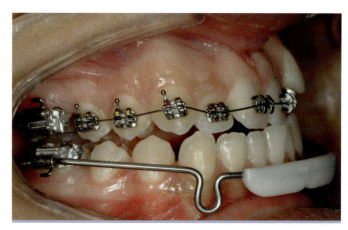

Figs 3.52, 3.53 & 3.54
Frontal and lateral views of the .014 round stainless steel archwire, with omega loops to the mesial of the molars to enable creation of space in the upper arch, and also resulting in labial tipping of the upper incisors. In the lower arch, the lip bumper is still in place.

Fig. 3.52

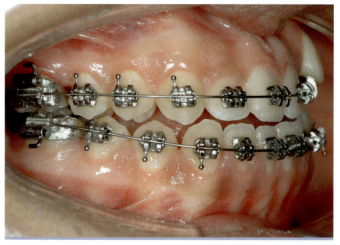

Figs 3.55, 3.56 & 3.57
Frontal and lateral views showing the .016 round Nitinol archwire in the upper arch with an open coil spring to open space for the upper left canine.

Fig. 3.55

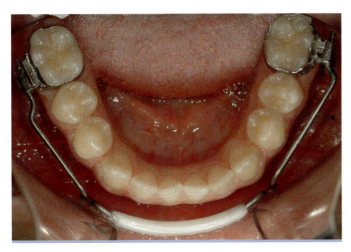

Fig. 3.51

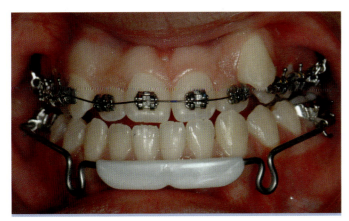

Fig. 3.53

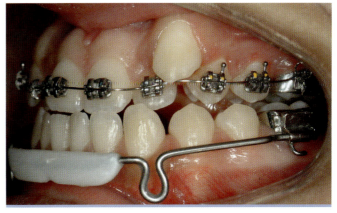

Fig. 3.54

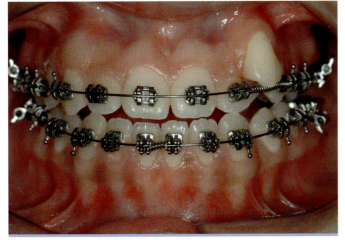

Fig. 3.56

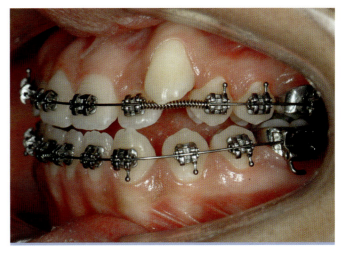

Fig. 3.57

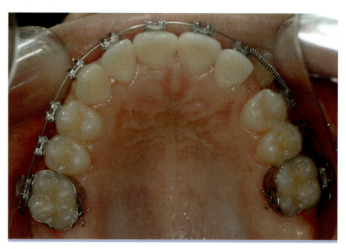

Fig. 3.58

Figs 3.58 & 3.59
Occlusal views showing the open coil spring. In the lower arch, spacing is observed in the premolar segment.

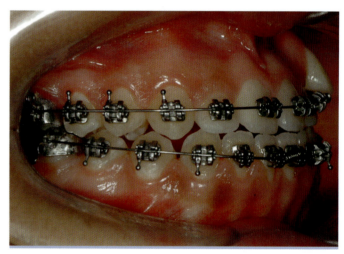

Fig. 3.60

Figs 3.60, 3.61 & 3.62
Frontal and lateral views, with .016 round stainless steel archwire and open coil spring and sufficient space gained for the upper left canine.

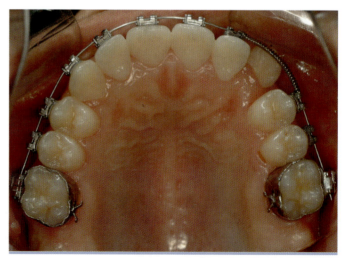

Fig. 3.63

Figs 3.63 & 3.64
Occlusal view showing a .016 round stainless steel archwire and adequate space for the upper left canine. The lower arch shows good form and spacing in the premolar area.

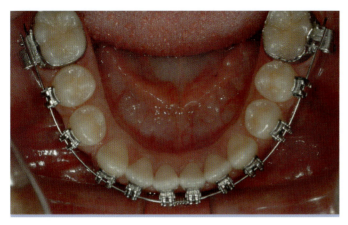

Fig. 3.59

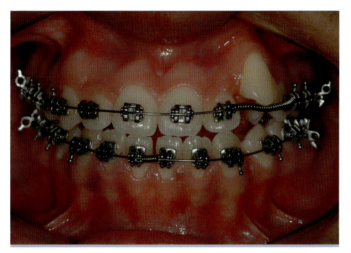

Fig. 3.61

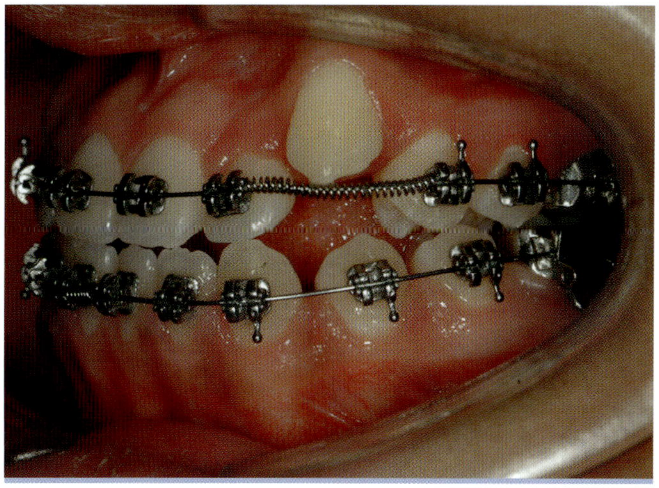

Fig. 3.62

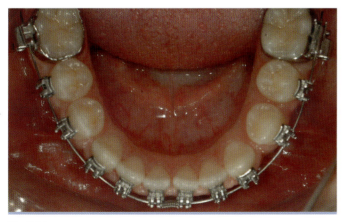

Fig. 3.64

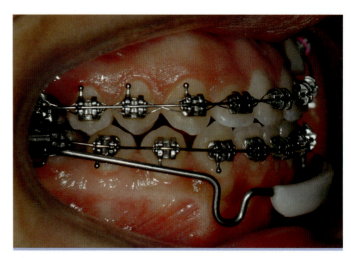

Fig. 3.65

Figs 3.65, 3.66 & 3.67
A .014 round Nitinol superelastic archwire engaged to initiate the alignment of the canine. In the lower arch, the .016 round stainless steel archwire and the lip bumper are in place.

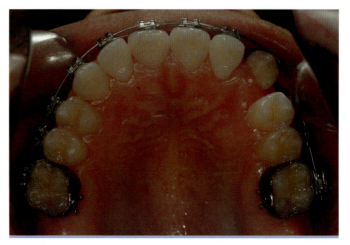

Fig. 3.68

Figs 3.68 & 3.69
Occlusal views again showing the space opened for the upper canine. The lower arch shows some spacing in the premolar area.

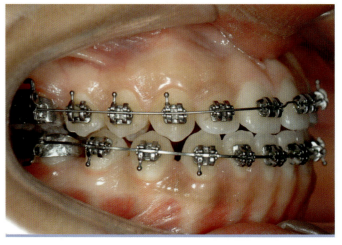

Fig. 3.70

Figs 3.70, 3.71 & 3.72
In the upper arch, a .016 round Nitinol superelastic archwire was engaged for final alignment of the upper left canine. In the lower arch, a .017/.025 rectangular Nitinol archwire was engaged to finalize the correction of the dental rotations.

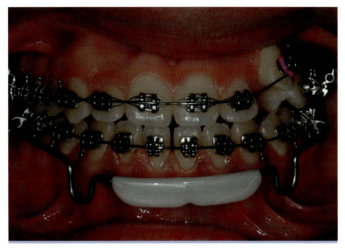

Fig. 3.66

Fig. 3.67

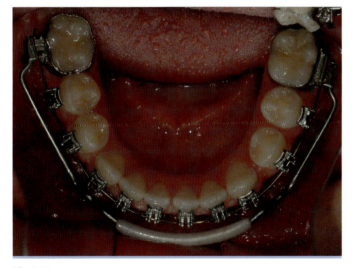

Fig. 3.69

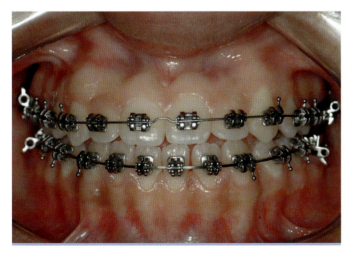

Fig. 3.71

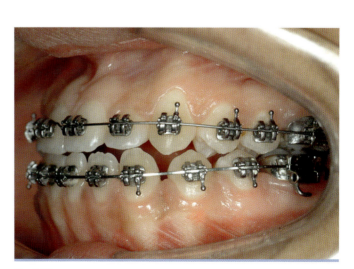

Fig. 3.72

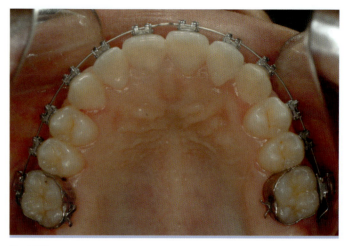

Fig. 3.73

Figs 3.73 & 3.74
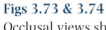
Occlusal views showing a .016 round Nitinol archwire and a .017/.025 rectangular archwire. A good arch form is seen in both dental arches.

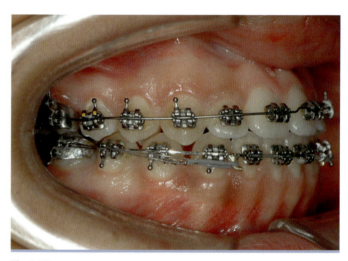

Fig. 3.75

Figs 3.75, 3.76 & 3.77
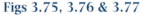
In the upper arch, a .016 round Nitinol superelastic archwire is in place and in the lower arch, a .019/.025 rectangular stainless steel archwire and .009 metal ligature with elastic modules attached from the first molars to the prewelded hook mesial to the canines.

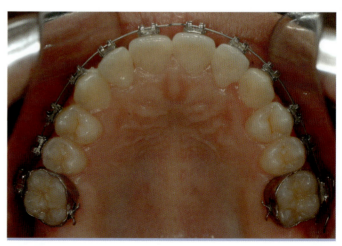

Fig. 3.78

Figs 3.78 & 3.79
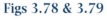
Occlusal views showing good dental arch form. In the lower dental arch, a .019/.025 rectangular stainless steel archwire was engaged for space closure. In this stage of treatment, the patient was asked to continue using the lip bumper.

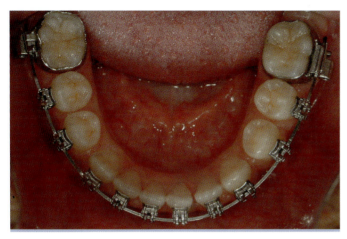

Fig. 3.74

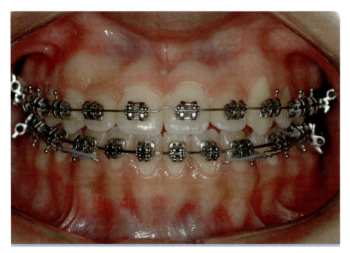

Fig. 3.76

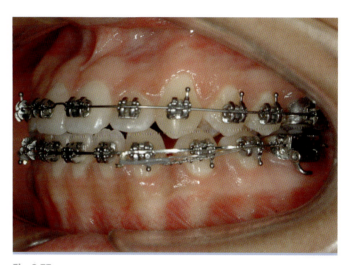

Fig. 3.77

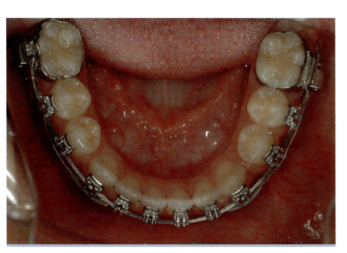

Fig. 3.79

Figs 3.80, 3.81 & 3.82
The .016 round Nitinol archwire still engaged in the upper arch while in the lower arch, the .019/.025 rectangular stainless steel was kept in place following space closure with passive tiebacks (.009 metal ligatures placed from the mesial of the molars to the prewelded hook to the mesial of the canines).

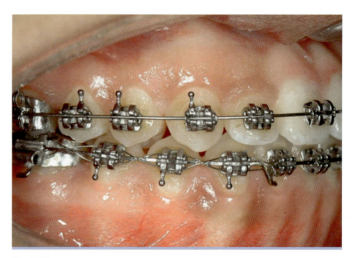

Fig. 3.80

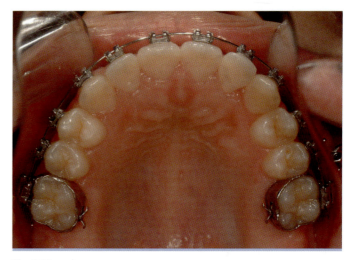

Fig. 3.83

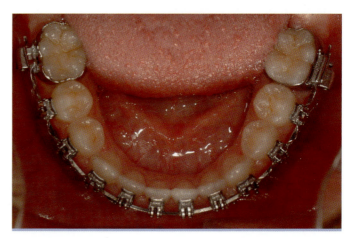

Figs 3.83 & 3.84
Occlusal views showing the .016 round Nitinol archwire in the upper arch and the .019/.025 rectangular stainless steel archwire in the lower arch with passive tiebacks to keep the spaces closed.

Fig. 3.84

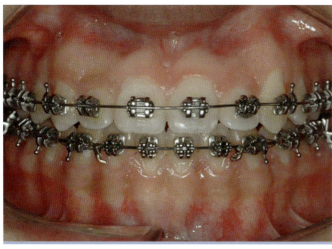

Fig. 3.81

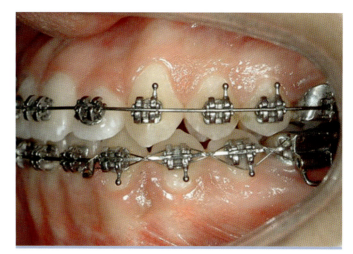

Fig. 3.82

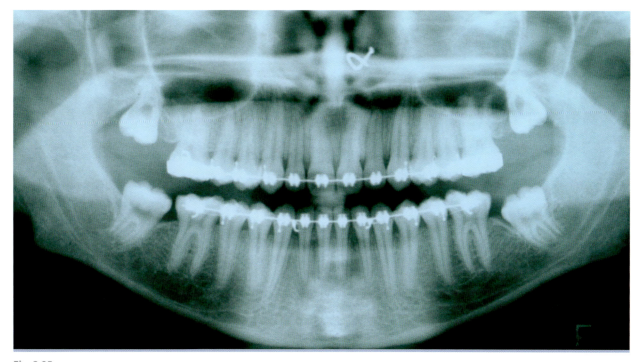

Fig. 3.85

Fig. 3.85
Panoramic radiograph showing good development, uprighting and eruption of the third molars toward the first molars.

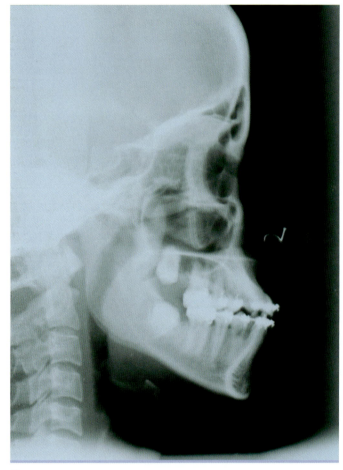

Fig. 3.86

Figs 3.86, 3.87 & 3.88
Cephalometric radiograph, tracing and analysis showing the correction of the anterior crossbite, with satisfactory compensation of the anterior tooth inclination.

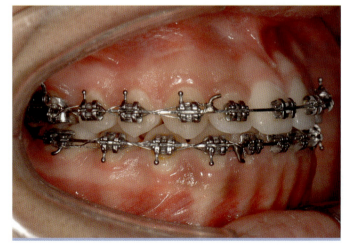

Fig. 3.89

Figs 3.89, 3.90 & 3.91
Frontal and lateral views showing a .019/.025 rectangular stainless steel archwire with passive tiebacks to hold the spaces closed. A good Class I molar relationship and adequate incisor overjet is seen.

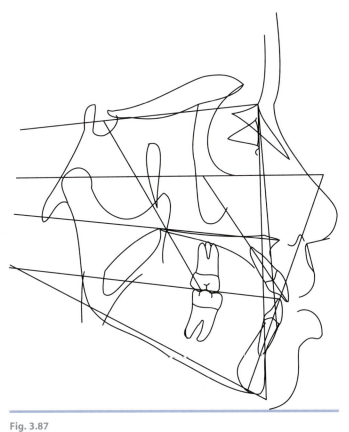

Fig. 3.87

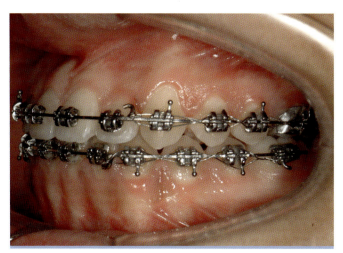

SNA ∠	89º
SNB ∠	86º
ANB ∠	3º
A-N ⊥ FH	4 mm
Po-N ⊥ FH	2 mm
Wits	–3 mm
GoGn SN ∠	32º
FH Md ∠	28º
Mx Md ∠	22º
U1 to A-Po	8 mm
L1 to A-Po	5 mm
U1 to Mx plane ∠	130º
L1 to Md plane ∠	82º
Facial analysis	
Nasolabial ∠	88º
NA ⊥ nose	28 mm
Lip thickness	11 mm

Fig. 3.88

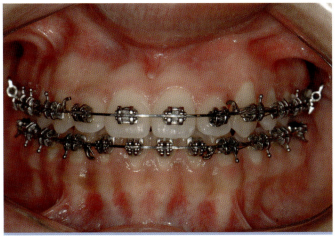

Fig. 3.90

Fig. 3.91

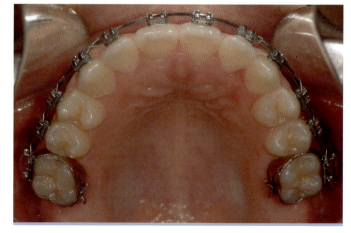

Fig. 3.92

Figs 3.92 & 3.93
Occlusal views after space closure showing good upper and lower dental arch forms and contact points.

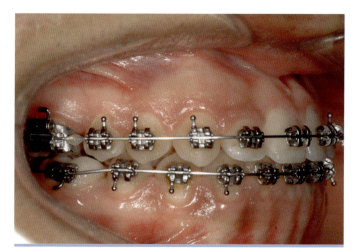

Fig. 3.94

Figs 3.94, 3.95 & 3.96
Bonded buccal tubes on the lower molars and bracket repositioning, with 180° bracket rotation, on the upper right lateral incisor for root torque and detailing of the occlusion. A .017/.025 rectangular Nitinol superelastic archwire was engaged for realignment.

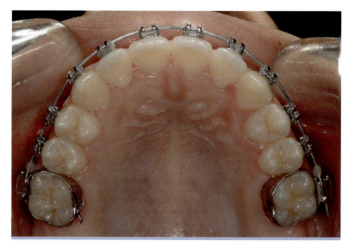

Fig. 3.97

Figs 3.97 & 3.98
Occlusal views after bonding the buccal tubes on the lower molars and repositioning of the upper left lateral incisor bracket, with .017/.025 rectangular archwires engaged.

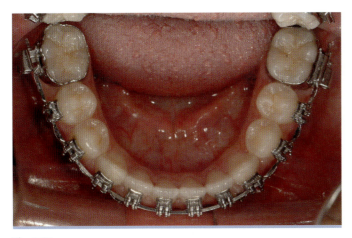

Fig. 3.93

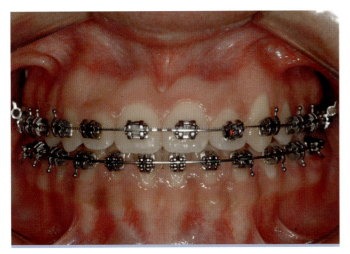

Fig. 3.95

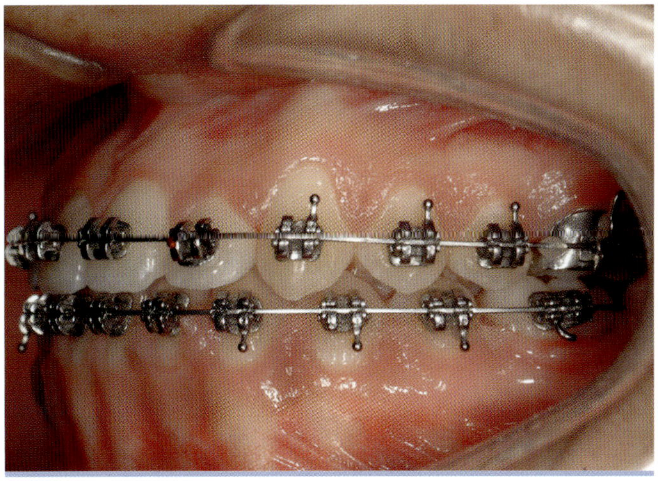

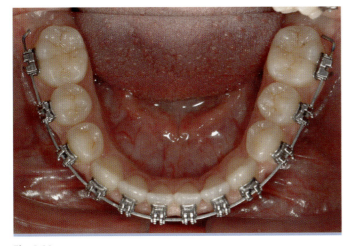

Fig. 3.96

Fig. 3.98

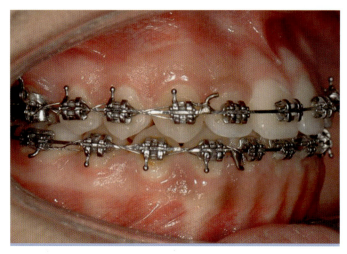

Figs 3.99, 3.100 & 3.101
Frontal and lateral views showing the final stage of the orthodontic treatment, with a .019/.025 rectangular stainless steel archwire and passive tiebacks from the molars to the prewelded hooks mesial to the canines. A good molar relationship, premolar intercuspation, canines in Class I relationship, and incisor overjet and overbite can be observed. The centerline discrepancy has been corrected.

Fig. 3.99

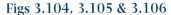

Figs 3.102 & 3.103
Occlusal views of the final stage of treatment with rectangular archwire. Good dental arch form and contact points are present.

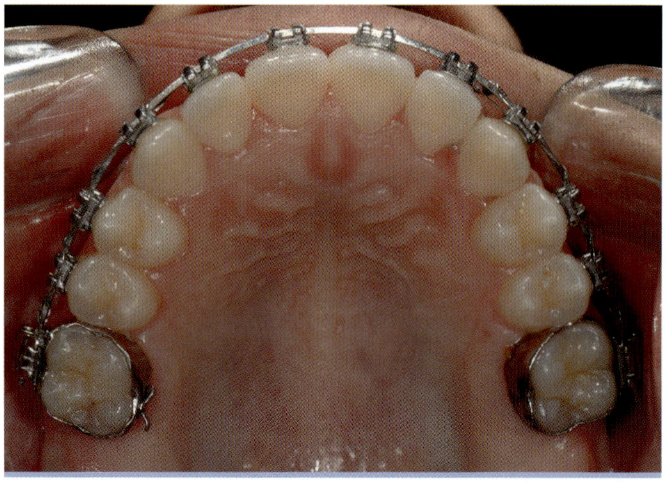

Fig. 3.102

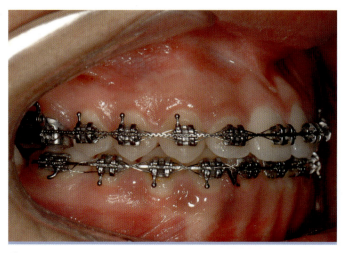

Figs 3.104, 3.105 & 3.106
Frontal and lateral views showing the finishing and detailing stages of treatment, with a .019/.025 rectangular braided archwire in the upper arch and a .019/.025 rectangular stainless steel archwire in the lower arch. A .009 ligature wire was placed under the braided archwire to prevent opening of spaces; 3/16 (4 oz) elastics were used to settle the occlusion.

Fig. 3.104

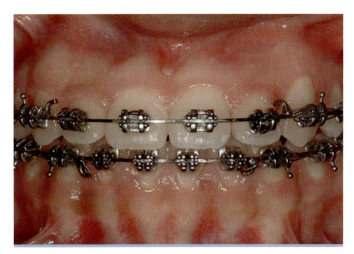

Fig. 3.100

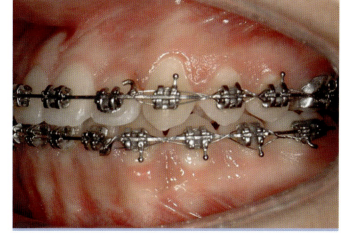

Fig. 3.101

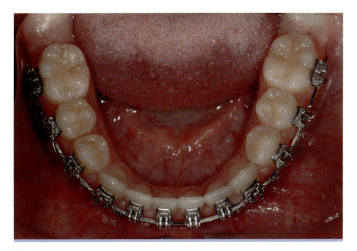

Fig. 3.103

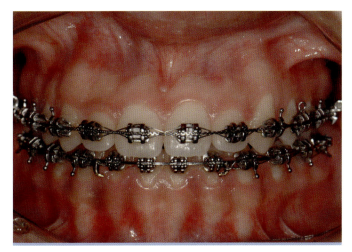

Fig. 3.105

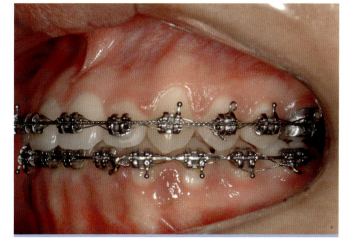

Fig. 3.106

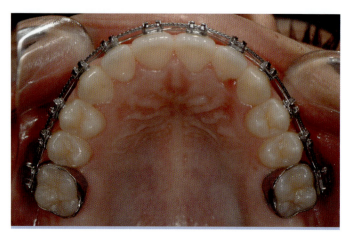

Figs 3.107 & 3.108

Occlusal views showing the upper dental arch with a braided archwire and the lower arch with a rectangular stainless steel archwire. The lower right third molar has started to erupt in contact with the first molar.

Fig. 3.107

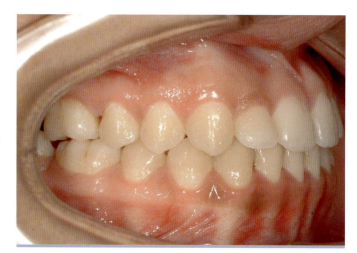

Figs 3.109, 3.110 & 3.111

Upper and lower appliance removal. The esthetic and functional goals of treatment have been achieved. There is a stable Class I molar and canine relationship, good overjet and incisor as well as canine overbite. The centerlines are corrected.

Fig. 3.109

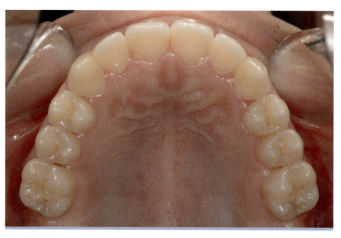

Figs 3.112 & 3.113

Occlusal views after upper and lower appliance removal showing good dental arch form and contact points. The lower right third molar has erupted in good contact with the first molar.

Fig. 3.112

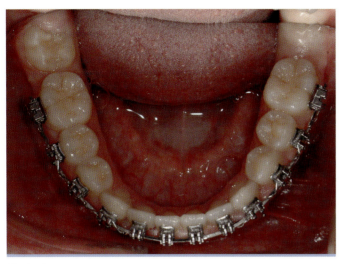

Fig. 3.108

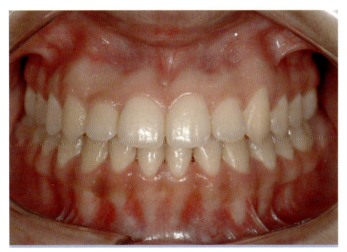

Fig. 3.110

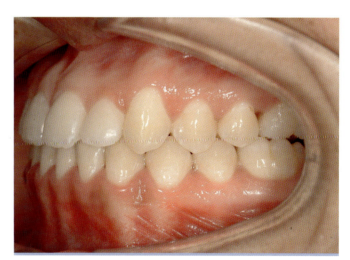

Fig. 3.111

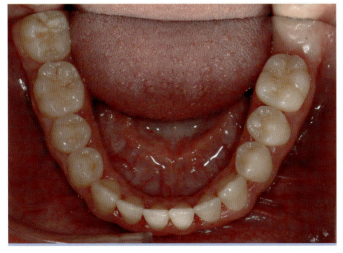

Fig. 3.113

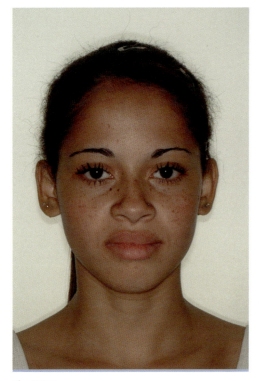

Fig. 3.114

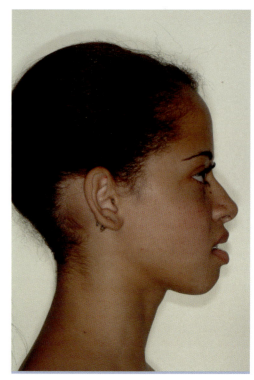

Fig. 3.115

Figs 3.114 & 3.115

Post-treatment extraoral photographs showing a very good treatment end result, with good facial harmony and lip seal.

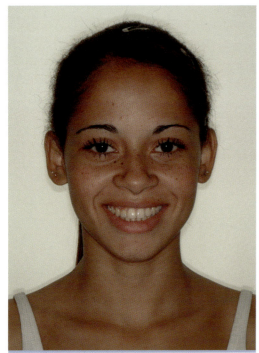

Fig. 3.116

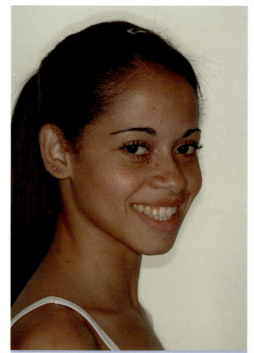

Fig. 3.117

Figs 3.116 & 3.117

Post-treatment extraoral photographs (frontal and 45°), showing a good smile line. The esthetic and functional goals have been achieved. The patient was very pleased with the end result of treatment.

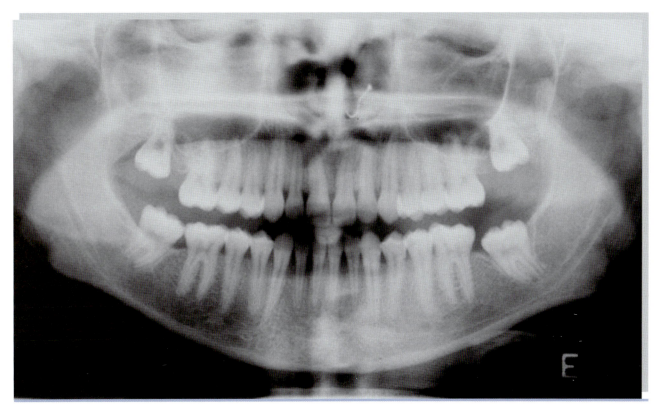

Fig. 3.118

Fig. 3.118
Panoramic radiograph after appliance removal. The third molars show good progress in eruption. The lower right third molar has erupted in contact with the first molar.

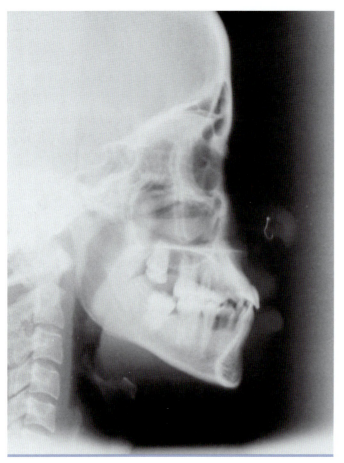

Fig. 3.119

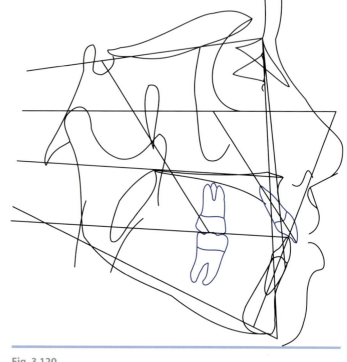

Fig. 3.120

Figs 3.119, 3.120 & 3.121
Cephalometric radiograph, tracing and analysis showing the treatment plan achieved the cephalometric goals established at the beginning of treatment.

SNA ∠	88º
SNB ∠	86º
ANB ∠	2º
A-N ⊥ FH	6 mm
Po-N ⊥ FH	6 mm
Wits	−2 mm
GoGn SN ∠	33º
FH Md ∠	26º
Mx Md ∠	22º
U1 to A-Po	8 mm
L1 to A-Po	5 mm
U1 to Mx plane ∠	126º
L1 to Md plane ∠	86º
Facial analysis	
Nasolabial ∠	98º
NA ⊥ nose	27 mm
Lip thickness	0 mm

Fig. 3.121

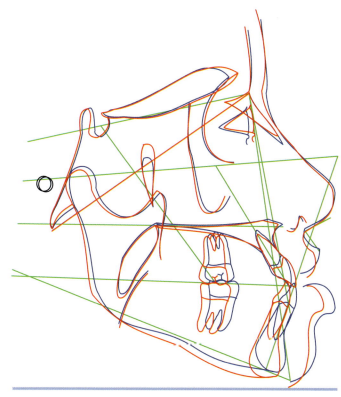

Fig. 3.122

Fig. 3.122
Superimposition of the initial and final tracing. There was good vertical and horizontal control, with correction of the overjet by alteration of the inclination of the upper and lower incisors.

Chapter 3 Clinical case 2

Name: JTS
Sex: Female
Age: 10 years, 7 months
Facial pattern: mesofacial
Skeletal pattern: Class II

Diagnosis

Class II skeletal malocclusion, Class II dental malocclusion on the right side, Class I dental malocclusion on the left side, upper incisors with labial rotation, upper and lower anterior crowding, accentuated curve of Spee, deep overbite and upper centerline deviation to the left side.

Treatment plan

Extraction of the upper right second molar, rapid maxillary expansion, expansion of the lower arch, distalization of the upper right first molar to achieve a Class I molar relationship, interarch relationship correction and upper centerline correction.

Appliances

- Hyrax expansion appliance in the upper arch
- Asymmetric headgear
- Fixed appliances in the upper and lower arches
- Class II elastics on the right side
- Hawley retainer in the upper arch
- 3 × 3 fixed retainer on the lower arch

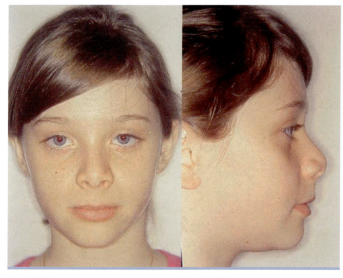

Fig. 3.123   Fig. 3.124

Figs 3.123 & 3.124
Pretreatment extraoral photographs showing facial symmetry and lip competence. The lateral view shows the Class II profile.

Case report

The treatment plan was to extract the upper right second molar to establish a Class I molar relationship, providing centerline correction, improve the interarch relationship and vertical and horizontal control of tooth movement during the orthodontic treatment phase.

Initially, a Hyrax appliance was placed with bands on the upper molars and premolars to expand the upper arch. A fixed appliance was bonded in the lower arch with a .014 round Nitinol archwire to commence the alignment. Shortly after the Hyrax appliance was removed, the upper right second molar was extracted and the asymmetric headgear used to distalize the first molar. The fixed appliance was set up with a .014 round Nitinol archwire.

After establishing the Class I molar relationship on the right side and finishing the upper and the lower alignment, .016, .018 and .020 round stainless steel archwires were engaged consecutively to complete leveling in both arches.

In the space closure stage of treatment, .019/.025 rectangular stainless steel archwires were engaged in both dental arches with passive tiebacks, which remained in place for a month. Subsequently, tooth retraction was carried out with metal ligatures and elastic modules. During this stage of treatment, extra buccal root torque was added to the incisal segment of the lower rectangular archwire with a reverse curve of Spee to correct the overbite.

In the final stage of treatment, a panoramic radiograph was taken to assess tooth alignment. A few brackets were repositioned and a minitube was bonded on the lower right second molar. A .016 round Nitinol archwire was engaged.

After re-leveling, a .019/.025 rectangular stainless steel archwire was engaged to complete the corrective treatment. The fixed appliances were removed after achieving perfect dental intercuspation and functional movements. Retention involved a Hawley retainer in the upper arch and a fixed 3 × 3 retainer in the lower arch.

A post-treatment panoramic radiograph was taken to check the eruption of the upper right third molar, which was seen to be in contact with the first molar. There was no need for further treatment to align and upright the upper right third molar.

The treatment achieved the functional and esthetic goals established at the beginning of treatment. The patient was very pleased with the end result of the orthodontic treatment.

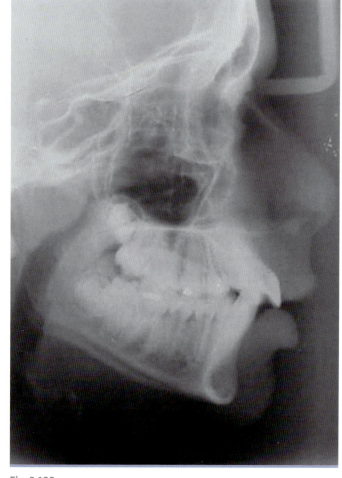

Figs 3.125, 3.126 & 3.127
Cephalometric radiograph, tracing and analysis showing the skeletal Class II relationship, Wits measurement of 8 mm and vertical measurements well balanced.

Fig. 3.125

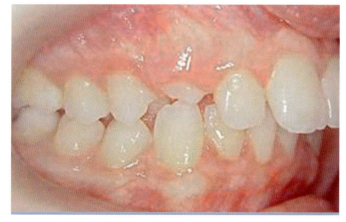

Figs 3.128, 3.129 & 3.130
Pretreatment intraoral photographs showing the Class II molar relationship on the right side and Class I molar relationship on the left side, a deep overbite and upper centerline deviation to the left.

Fig. 3.128

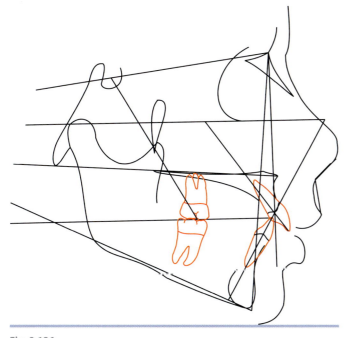

Fig. 3.126

SNA ∠	82º
SNB ∠	75º
ANB ∠	7º
A-N ⊥ FH	1 mm
Po-N ⊥ FH	−7 mm
Wits	8 mm
GoGn SN ∠	35º
FH Md ∠	26º
Mx Md ∠	22º
U1 to A-Po	9 mm
L1 to A-Po	2 mm
U1 to Mx plane ∠	129º
L1 to Md plane ∠	93º
Facial analysis	
Nasolabial ∠	127º
NA ⊥ nose	26 mm
Lip thickness	12 mm

Fig. 3.127

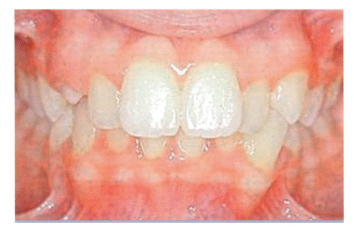

Fig. 3.129

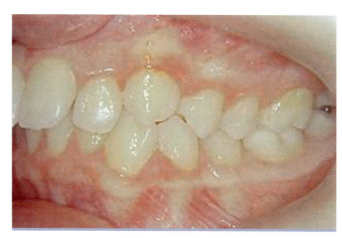

Fig. 3.130

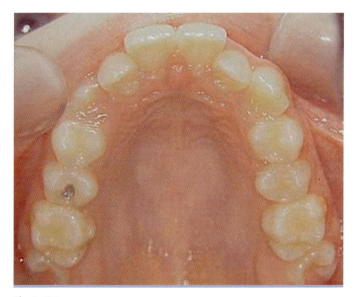

Fig. 3.131

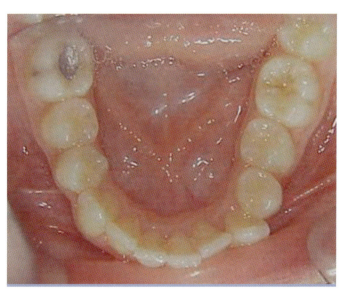

Figs 3.131 & 3.132
Occlusal views showing narrow dental arches and crowding in both upper and lower dental arches.

Fig. 3.132

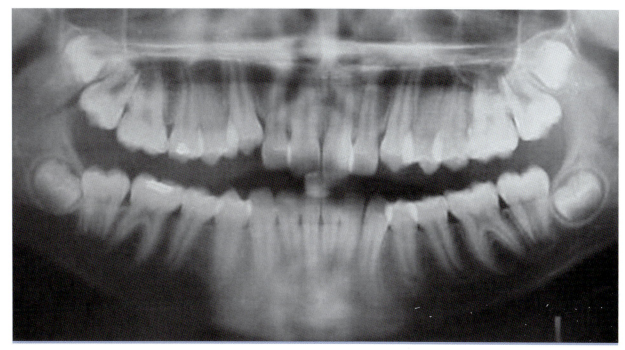

Fig. 3.133

Fig. 3.133
Panoramic radiograph showing developing third molars of good shape and size.

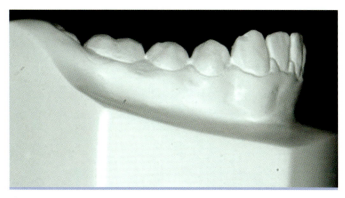

Fig. 3.134

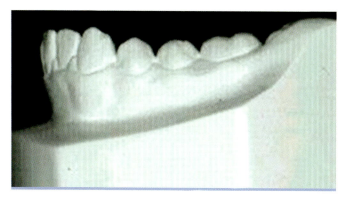

Fig. 3.135

Figs 3.134 & 3.135
Lateral views of the lower arch study model showing the increased curve of Spee.

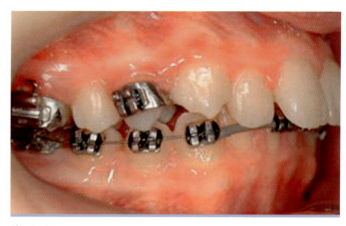

Fig. 3.136

Figs 3.136, 3.137 & 3.138
Frontal and lateral views of the Hyrax appliance with bands on the first molars and the first premolars. Appliance set-up in the lower arch with a .014 round Nitinol archwire in the beginning of the alignment stage.

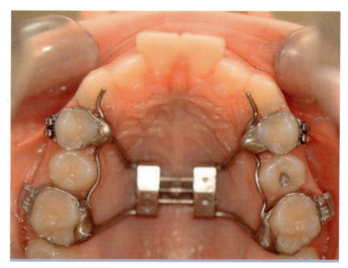

Fig. 3.139

Figs 3.139 & 3.140
Occlusal views showing rapid maxillary expansion being carried out and appliance set-up on the lower arch with .014 round Nitinol archwire.

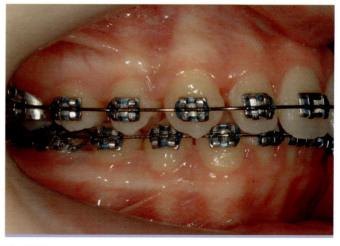

Fig. 3.141

Figs 3.141, 3.142 & 3.143
Frontal and lateral views with .016 round stainless steel archwire initiating the leveling stage in the lower arch. After the extraction of the upper right second molar, the upper right first molar was in a Class I relationship. The patient was using the headgear and the median diastema seen is due to previous rapid maxillary expansion.

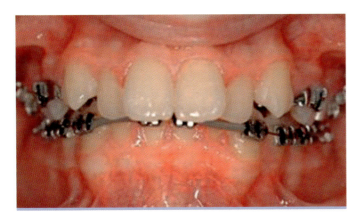

Fig. 3.137

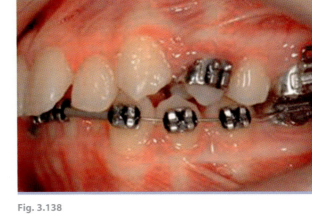

Fig. 3.138

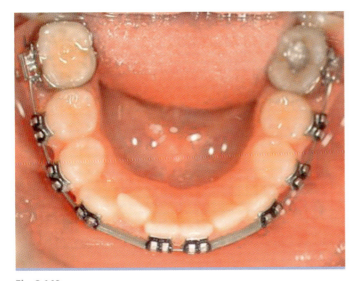

Fig. 3.140

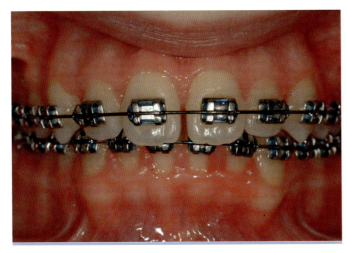

Fig. 3.142

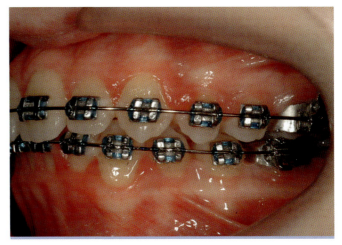

Fig. 3.143

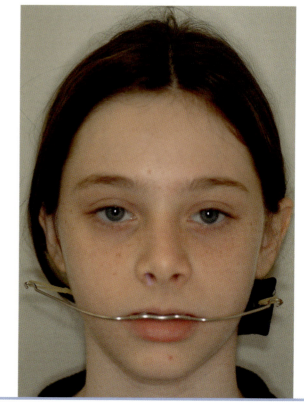

Figs 3.144 & 3.145
Frontal and lateral views of the patient with the asymmetric headgear in place for distalizing the upper right molar.

Fig. 3.144

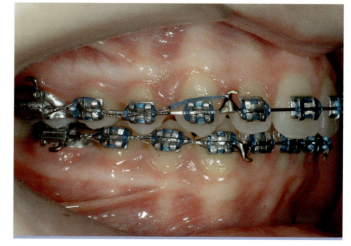

Figs 3.146, 3.147 & 3.148
Frontal and lateral views with .019/.025 rectangular stainless steel archwire and passive tiebacks placed from the prewelded hook mesial to the canines to the molars.

Fig. 3.146

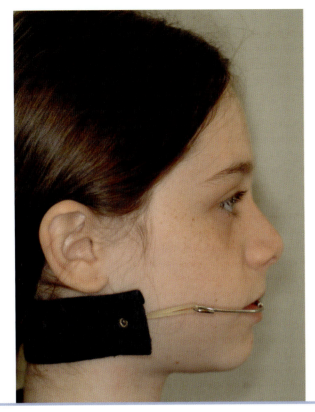

Fig. 3.145

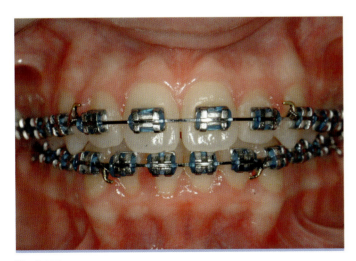

Fig. 3.147

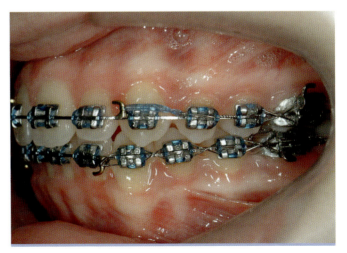

Fig. 3.148

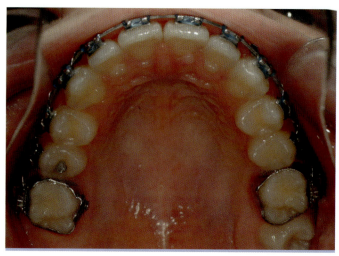

Figs 3.149 & 3.150

Occlusal views of the fixed appliances in place with .019/.025 rectangular stainless steel archwires.

Fig. 3.149

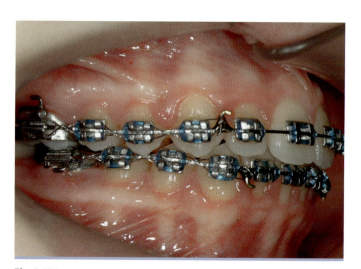

Figs 3.151, 3.152 & 3.153

Frontal and lateral views with .019/.025 rectangular stainless steel archwires in place. Retraction mechanics are being applied, using metal ligatures and elastic modules placed from the molar to the prewelded hook to the mesial of the canines.

Fig. 3.151

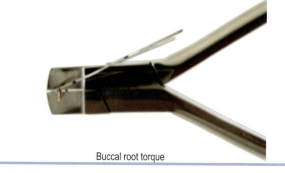

Figs 3.154 & 3.155

Figure 3.154 shows the introduction of buccal root torque to the .019/.025 rectangular archwire for the lower incisors, and Figure 3.155 shows the archwire with reverse curve in the lower archwire for correcting the overbite and at the same time preventing the lower incisor tipping buccally.

Buccal root torque

Fig. 3.154

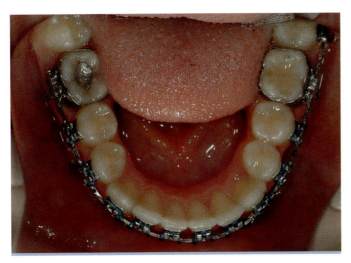

Fig. 3.150

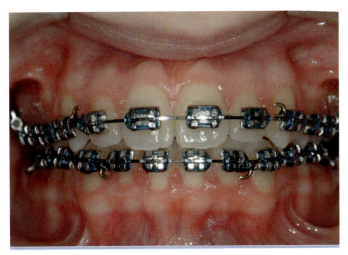

Fig. 3.152

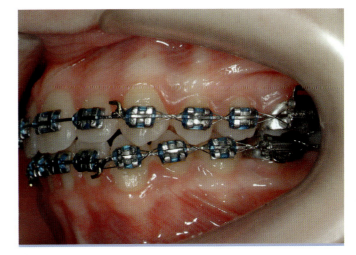

Fig. 3.153

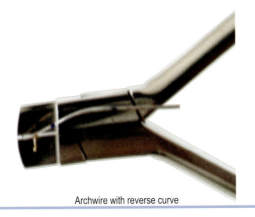

Archwire with reverse curve

Fig. 3.155

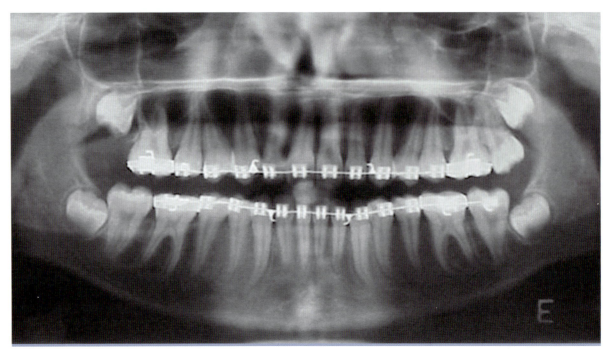

Fig. 3.156

Fig. 3.156
Interim panoramic radiograph to verify the root positioning and the progress in eruption of the upper right third molar.

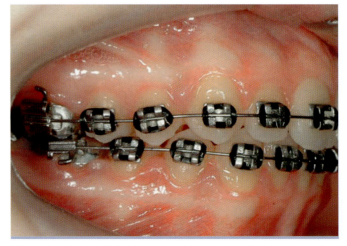

Figs 3.160, 3.161 & 3.162
Frontal and lateral views showing the engagement of .016 round Nitinol archwire after bracket repositioning.

Fig. 3.160

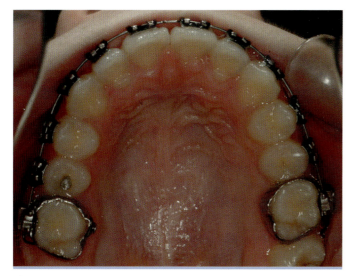

Fig. 3.157

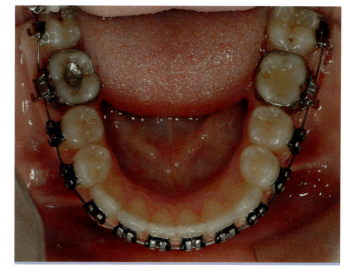

Fig. 3.158

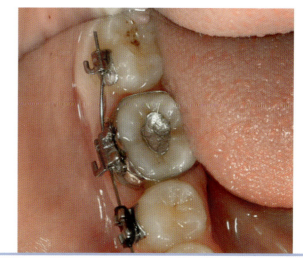

Fig. 3.159

Figs 3.157, 3.158 & 3.159
Occlusal views showing the .016 round Nitinol archwire in the upper arch after bracket repositioning. Figure 3.159 shows the minitube bonded to the lower right second molar.

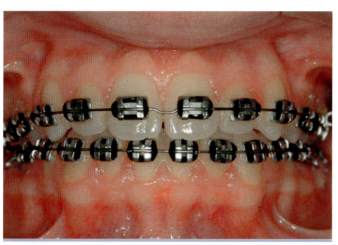

Fig. 3.161

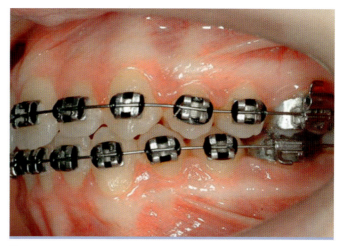

Fig. 3.162

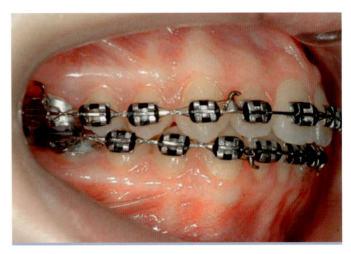

Figs 3.163, 3.164 & 3.165

Frontal and lateral views with .019/.025 rectangular stainless steel archwire and passive tiebacks from the molars to the prewelded hook to the mesial of the canines in the final stage of treatment.

Fig. 3.163

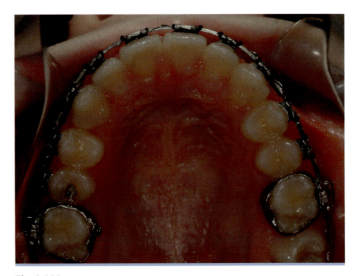

Figs 3.166 & 3.167

Occlusal views of the .019/.025 rectangular stainless steel archwires in the final stage of treatment. There is good arch form and alignment with contact points well established in both arches.

Fig. 3.166

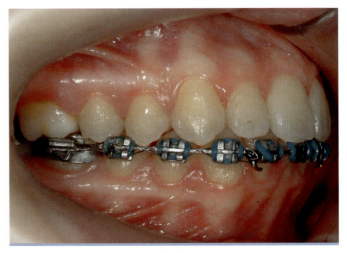

Figs 3.168, 3.169 & 3.170

Frontal and lateral views after upper appliance removal with centerline corrected and Class I molar relationship. In the lower arch, the fixed appliance was kept in place with a .019/.025 rectangular archwire for 1 more month.

Fig. 3.168

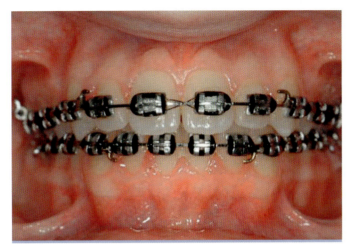

Fig. 3.164

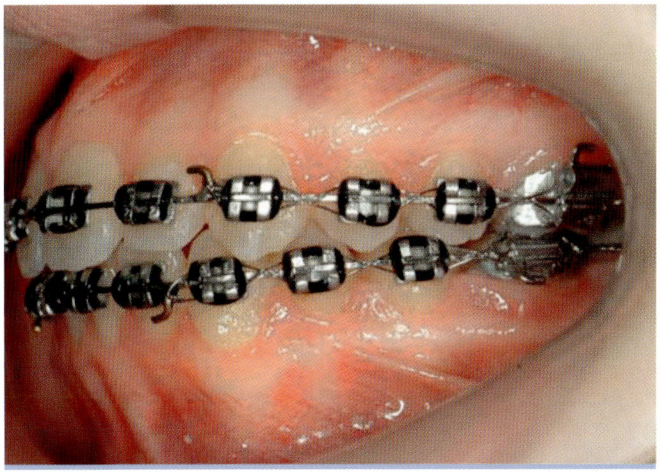

Fig. 3.165

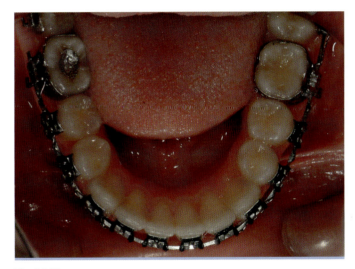

Fig. 3.167

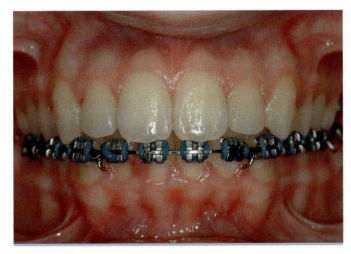

Fig. 3.169

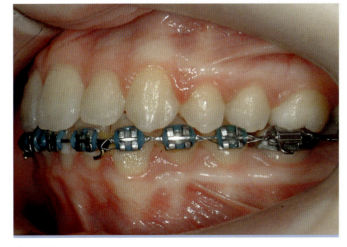

Fig. 3.170

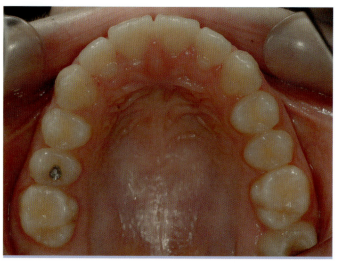

Fig. 3.171

Figs 3.171 & 3.172

Occlusal views showing the upper arch after fixed appliance removal. The fixed lower appliance is still in place.

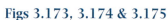

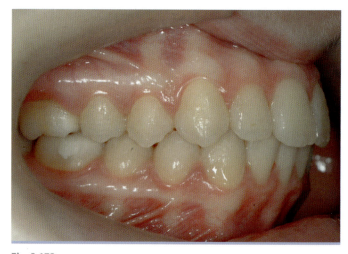

Fig. 3.173

Figs 3.173, 3.174 & 3.175

Frontal and lateral views after fixed appliance removal. The functional and esthetic goals of the orthodontic treatment were achieved. The molar relationship and the upper centerline were corrected and overjet and overbite well established.

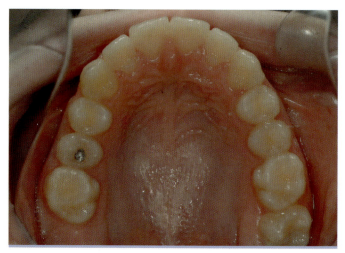

Fig. 3.176

Figs 3.176 & 3.177

Occlusal view of both upper and lower dental arches showing good dental arch form. In the upper arch, the upper right third molar is still not erupted. In the lower arch there is a fixed 3 × 3 retainer fabricated from .018 twist-flex archwire.

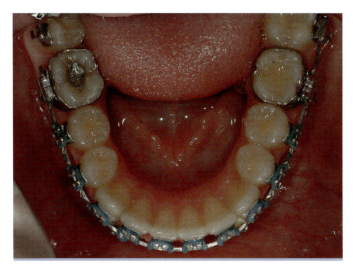

Fig. 3.172

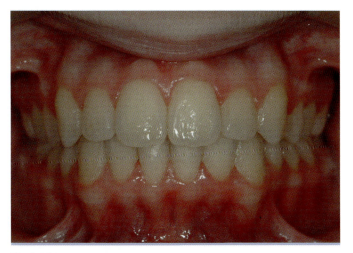

Fig. 3.174

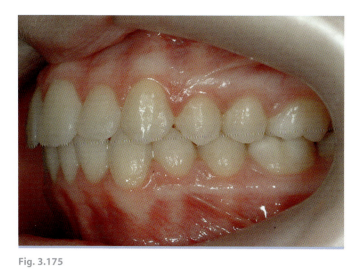

Fig. 3.175

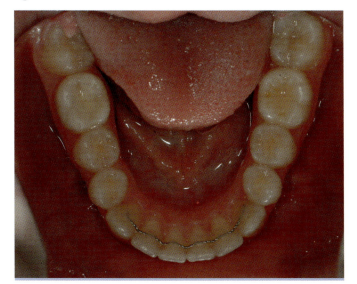

Fig. 3.177

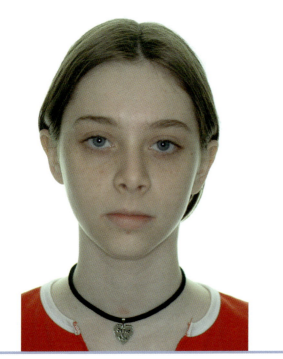

Fig. 3.178

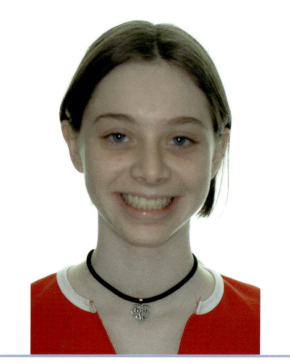

Fig. 3.179

Figs 3.178 & 3.179
Post-treatment extraoral photographs showing good facial esthetics and harmony and smile line.

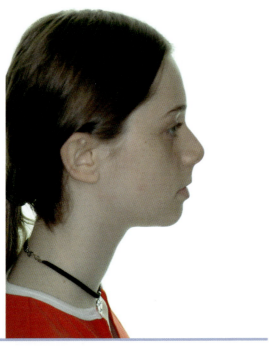

Fig. 3.180

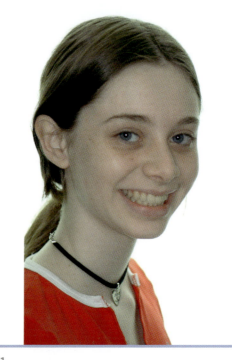

Fig. 3.181

Figs 3.180 & 3.181
Post-treatment extraoral photographs showing a good smile line. The functional and esthetic treatment goals were achieved. The patient was pleased with the treatment outcome.

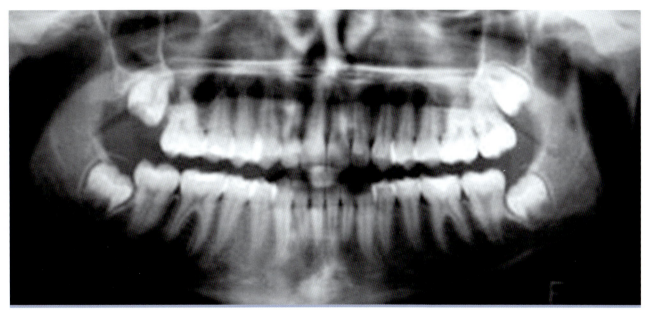

Fig. 3.182

Fig. 3.182
Panoramic radiograph after the appliance removal confirming good progress in the eruption of the upper right third molar.

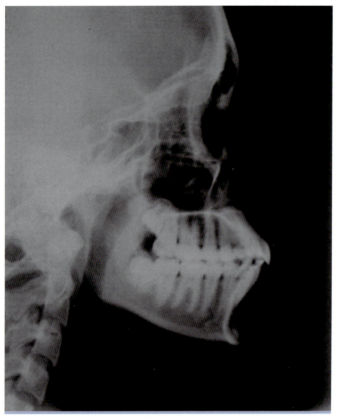

Fig. 3.183

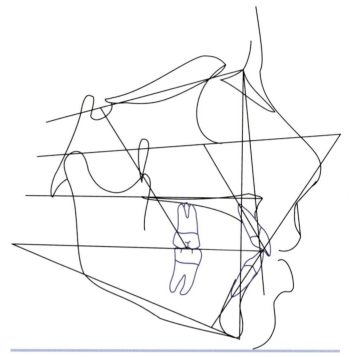

Fig. 3.184

Figs 3.183, 3.184 & 3.185
Cephalometric radiograph, tracing and analysis confirming that the treatment achieved the goals established at the beginning of treatment.

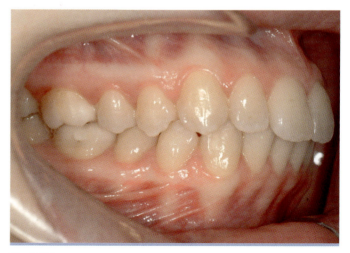

Figs 3.187, 3.188 & 3.189
Extraoral photographs 1 year after the treatment was completed. The molar relationship was stable and the third molar erupted in good contact with the first molar.

Fig. 3.187

SNA ∠	81°
SNB ∠	75°
ANB ∠	6°
A-N ⊥ FH	2 mm
Po-N ⊥ FH	–7 mm
Wits	6 mm
GoGn SN ∠	35°
FH Md ∠	26°
Mx Md ∠	21°
U1 to A-Po	8 mm
L1 to A-Po	5 mm
U1 to Mx plane ∠	122°
L1 to Md plane ∠	103°
Facial analysis	
Nasolabial ∠	129°
NA ⊥ nose	30 mm
Lip thickness	11 mm

Fig. 3.185

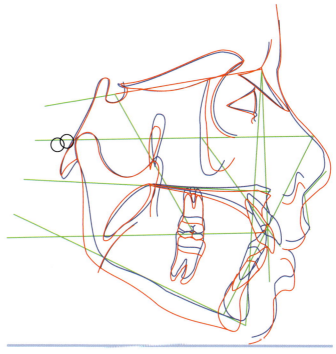

Fig. 3.186

Fig. 3.186

Superimposition of the initial and the final tracings. There was a good vertical and horizontal control allowing the correction of the overjet. The lower incisors were positioned according to the dental VTO set out at the beginning of the treatment.

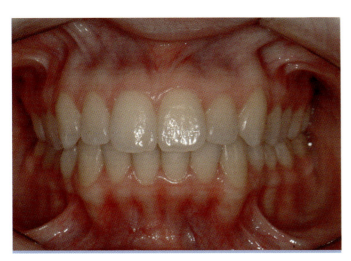

Fig. 3.188

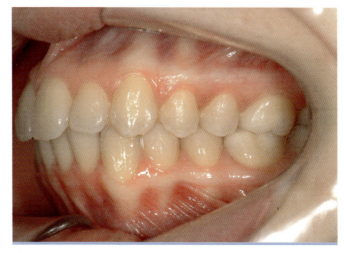

Fig. 3.189

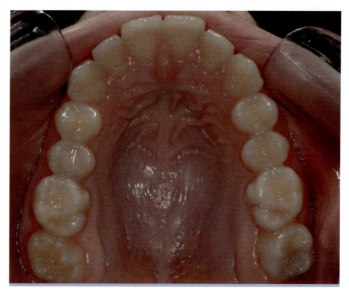

Fig. 3.190

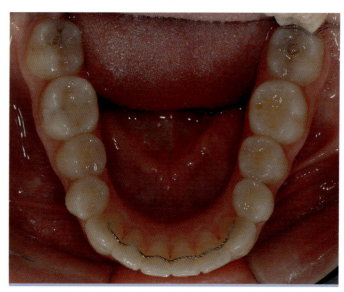

Figs 3.190 & 3.191
Occlusal views of the upper and the lower dental arches. The upper right third molar has erupted in good contact with the first molar, without the need for further treatment.

Fig. 3.191

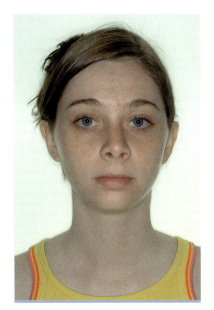
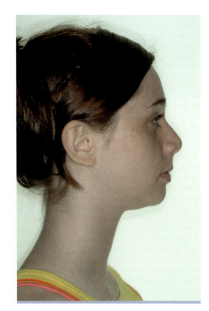

Fig. 3.192

Fig. 3.193

Figs 3.192 & 3.193
Frontal and profile photographs showing good lip competence.

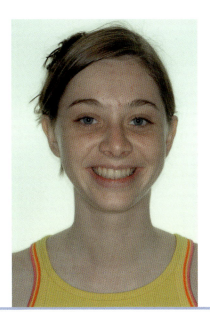

Fig. 3.194

Fig. 3.194
Frontal smiling photograph showing good esthetics. The patient was pleased with the final treatment result.

Index